The future
public health

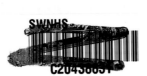

The future public health

Phil Hanlon, Sandra Carlisle,
Margaret Hannah and Andrew Lyon

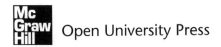 Open University Press

Open University Press
McGraw-Hill Education
McGraw-Hill House
Shoppenhangers Road
Maidenhead
Berkshire
England
SL6 2QL

email: enquiries@openup.co.uk
world wide web: www.openup.co.uk

and Two Penn Plaza, New York, NY 10121-2289, USA

First published 2012

A catalogue record of this book is available from the British Library

ISBN-13: 9780335243556 (pb)
ISBN-10: 033524355x (pb)
e-ISBN: 9780335243587

Library of Congress Cataloging-in-Publication Data
CIP data has been applied for

Typeset by Aptara Inc., India

Printed and bound by CPI Group (UK) Ltd, Croydon, CR0 4YY

Fictitous names of companies, products, people, characters and/or data that may be used herein (in case studies or in examples) are not intended to represent any real individual, company, product or event.

The McGraw·Hill Companies

Praise for this book

"Health is created in the context of everyday life. This book helps us understand what this means in the 21st century and how public health must be reframed to respond effectively. It grounds the new approach to public health in systems thinking, challenges mantras of modernity and prioritizes sustainability and well being. Read it and take the third public health revolution the next step forward."

Professor Ilona Kickbusch, Director Global Health Programme,
The Graduate Institute, Geneva, Switzerland

"This excellent book could not be more timely. It must now be apparent to almost everyone that we cannot go on as we have done in the past, believing that we can consume an ever greater amount of the earth's limited resources and somehow it will all work out. It won't. By painting a picture on a broad canvas, the authors set out a vision of a future in which we have rebalanced our relationship with the world around us. They give us a sense of purpose and reason for hope that, together, we might be able to attain it."

Professor Martin McKee CBE, London School of Hygiene and
Tropical Medicine, UK

"With the emerging evidence from the Human Genome Project that genes play little part in the genesis of most illness, this is a particularly timely book: it shows the central part that public health interventions must play in creating a healthy population."

Oliver James, Broadcaster, journalist, clinical psychologist and
bestselling book author

Contents

PART 3
The future public health

List of boxes

List of figures

List of tables

Foreword

I admire Phil Hanlon, Sandra Carlisle, Margaret Hannah and Andrew Lyon, not just for the lucidity with which they write, but for having the courage to question current public health practice and the creativity to suggest how things might change for the better in the future. Perhaps their diverse backgrounds, their experience of working in other parts of the globe and in a myriad of different capacities in the UK, have enabled them to look radically at our current situation and, at the same time, keep their feet firmly on the ground.

There can be no question that they are right in their basic assumption that things cannot go on as they are, either in public health or in society at large. In public health we are failing to make significant inroads into the key issues of our era: persisting social inequalities in health, obesity, addiction related harm, iatrogenic disease and the reducing rate of return on investment in the health service. The societies whose health we work to improve are going to have to change radically to cope with peak oil, climate change and an outdated economic framework based on continuing growth.

One of the functions of public health is to envision a different future; one in which current health problems can be avoided and health can improve. But sometimes old patterns of thinking get in the way of the radical solutions needed. Short termism, encouraged by our political masters, and reductionist thinking, encouraged by the current scientific paradigm, are the enemies of creativity and insight.

Hanlon and his co-authors outline the different eras in public health and the shifts in thinking that enabled movement from one to the other. They go on to outline ideas for future public health that represent a radical departure from the present. They investigate well-being and show how our current way of life in the western world, based on consumerism, individualism, competitiveness and the workplace treadmill, does not lend itself to well-being. The things that make for well-being – uncommitted time, pleasure in others' company, creative endeavour and giving to others – are the things we tend to squeeze out.

The authors instead propose a new way of thinking about public health, based on systems approaches, which are at heart holistic and integrative. In doing so they recognize that Cartesian thinking is well past its sell by date. We cannot go on pretending that the mind and body operate independently or that neither is affected by the state of our spirits. We must find a way of thinking and planning that takes into account their fundamental interrelatedness. To do so we need to embrace complexity theory and other now well established scientific paradigms that are not taught as part of the public health curriculum.

Hanlon and co-authors suggest framing our thinking in terms of the integration of 'the good, the true and the beautiful' or ethics, science and art. They may not have all the answers. There may be other frameworks we should also consider, but their book will have done its job if we find the courage to move outside our comfort zones and engage in thinking radically about these issues. It will also have done its job if we understand that we need to engage all of ourselves in that thinking not just the logical, cognitive brain with whose solutions we tend to feel so comfortable.

Sarah Stewart-Brown
Professor of Public Health, Warwick Medical School

Acknowledgements

This book derives from work funded by the National Programme for Improving Mental Health and Well-being in Scotland, i.e. the Culture and Well-being in Scotland research project. We would especially like to thank Geoff Huggins, Head of the Mental Health Division of the Scottish Government, for his efforts in securing that funding over an extended period. We have also been actively supported by the Glasgow Centre for Population Health and its director, Professor Carol Tannahill.

Thanks are due to members of our research steering group, in particular Dr David Reilly, Medical Director of the Centre for Integrative Care in Glasgow, whose inspirational work in reorienting medical care has informed our thinking over many years. Other members of the group, past and present, include Gregor Henderson, Lauren Murdoch, Stephanie Young and Mary Morton.

The International Futures Forum, based in Scotland, has also provided a source of fresh thinking on the 'change of age' now facing humanity. Their contribution to this work is not so much in this or that aspect of the arguments we set out, but rather in the way that the whole problem is seen. We would like to acknowledge, in particular, Graham Leicester, Maureen O'Hara, Bill Sharpe and Tony Hodgson.

Contributors

Phil Hanlon was educated in the West of Scotland and graduated in medicine from Glasgow University in 1978. Following a period of clinical experience in adult medicine and general practice he took up a research post with the Medical Research Council in the Gambia, West Africa. On returning to the UK he completed a period of training in public health after which he was appointed to the post of Director of Health Promotion for the Greater Glasgow Health Board. In 1994 he became a senior lecturer in public health at the University of Glasgow and was promoted to Professor in 1999. Between January 2001 and April 2003 Phil undertook a secondment to establish the Public Health Institute of Scotland, before returning to full-time academic life as Professor of Public Health at the University of Glasgow. Since then he has been involved in numerous research projects; his research interests include the uses of integrated public health data and evaluation of complex public health interventions. Phil has led the Culture and Well-being study (funded by the Scottish Government) since its inception in 2005. As part of this work he has become actively engaged in developing new forms of 'thinking, being and doing' for public health. He is the driving force behind a new website (www.afternow.co.uk) which poses the question, 'what's next for the health of society?' In this book he and his co-authors seek to provide some answers.

Sandra Carlisle was born in Wallasey in 1954 but did not get around to going to university until 1990. As a mature student at Keele University she studied English language and literature, and medical social anthropology and sociology: the latter led to a lifelong love of research in this field, applied to public health. As an even more mature student she gained her PhD at the University of Edinburgh. Over the years she has been involved in numerous public health and policy-related research and evaluation projects in academic and voluntary sector settings. A committed serial contract researcher, she counts herself extremely lucky to have been able to work on a whole range of intellectually fascinating and personally engaging research projects. She is now based in the Public Health Section at the University of Glasgow, working with Professor Phil Hanlon on an exploration of the relationship between 'modern' culture and well-being, and the implications for public health. Much of her work is accessible through the website (www.afternow.co.uk) where she and her colleagues hope to share their findings and insights with the public health community and interested others.

Andrew Lyon was born in Kilmarnock in 1954. He left school at 16, working in a tailor's shop and then a hi-fi store before becoming a carpet weaver in 1973. He studied sociology and economics at Edinburgh University 1976–80. He conducted research for his PhD in India between 1981 and 1983 and again in 1985. In 1986 he became coordinator of the Glasgow Healthy Cities Project, part of the World Health Organization (WHO) Europe programme. During this period he also acted as a consultant for WHO in Europe and Bangladesh. He became acting Chief Executive of Forward Scotland, the sustainable development charity, in 2000. In 2001 he joined the International Futures Forum (IFF) as 'Converger': the IFF is a non-profit organization, established to support transformative responses to complex and confounding challenges, and to restore our capacity for effective action in a change of age (see www.internationalfuturesforum.co.uk). Andrew has engaged in voluntary activity for most of his adult life, including a spell as the Scottish Director of Sustrans, the cycle path charity. He was, until recently, a founding director at Common Wheel, a charity which helped rehabilitating mental health patients to recycle bicycles at prices people can afford. Currently he is a director of Community Renewal, a charity which supports people living in deprived circumstances to fulfil their aspirations, and of AdHom, a medical charity based in Glasgow. He has also worked as honorary lecturer in Public Health at the University of Glasgow. He is a founder member of the advisory group for the Culture and Well-being study and has facilitated that group's many 'learning journeys' across Scottish society. He is a co-author of the website, www.afternow.co.uk. In his spare time, he says he can play the flute and the uilleann pipes: his children say he can't. In fair weather, he is an enthusiastic but poor amateur astronomer and likes to cycle whenever he can.

Margaret Hannah has been working in Fife, Scotland for 14 years, most recently as Deputy Director of Public Health. Her main areas of responsibility are in health protection and service re-design. She has been interested in health inequalities ever since she learnt about them as a medical student. The more she studied them, the more convinced she was that she should go into public health! Margaret was part of the Healthy Public Policy Network from its inception. The network has published *The Possible Scot* and a number of subsequent reports, including *The Fifth Wave: Searching for Health in Scotland*. Her strong links with the International Futures Forum in Aberdour (www.internationalfuturesforum.co.uk) have shaped her thinking in recent years and she now works as a member of IFF to promote the Fifth Wave. She was also a founding member of the advisory group for the Culture and Well-being study and co-author of the website, www.afternow.co.uk.

Part 1

Public health past and present

1 Towards the future public health

Introduction

The purpose of this book is to explain the need for, and begin to articulate a vision of, the future public health and its practitioners. As a discipline, public health is concerned with protecting, preserving and promoting the health of people living now *and* the health of generations yet unborn. The public health community is also concerned with the conditions that create or damage health, and has no real difficulty with the idea that the nature of present-day society can have far-reaching impacts on the health of future generations. In this respect, therefore, public health is about taking action today to protect and promote health and well-being tomorrow (Graham 2010). Yet public health research and practice is largely oriented towards the present and near future: as such, we are 'prisoners of the proximate' (McMichael 1999). The concentration on immediate risks and short term benefits for health accords well with today's needs and with a contemporary political discourse which emphasizes personal responsibility for health (Graham 2010). However, it accords poorly with a focus on the conditions for health, well-being and the sustainability of human society in the future (Hanlon and Carlisle 2010).

It is as well to spell out at this stage what this book is not: it is not an introductory text to public health or health promotion. Excellent books which serve this purpose already exist (e.g. Naidoo and Wills 2000; Pencheon et al. 2001; Pomerleau and Mckee 2005; Orme et al. 2007; McDowell et al. 2007; Donaldson and Scally 2009). Rather, this text presents a new way of understanding some of the key challenges confronting the discipline of public health in a rapidly changing, unstable and unpredictable world. It is based on a set of critical arguments about the nature of those challenges; arguments which are themselves underpinned by a growing body of evidence (Hanlon et al. 2011). This body of evidence and the conclusions to which it leads are rarely brought together in one place for the public health community. The book can therefore be understood as a first attempt to bridge the gap between the values and skills that currently inform this discipline and those that will be needed to face the future. No blueprints for the future exist. However, this book could help colleagues across the broad constituency of public health (including students and established practitioners) to address the urgent challenge of discovering the potential for positive change in an increasingly difficult environment. This chapter briefly outlines the widely varying nature of the new public health challenges. It begins to make the case for a radically different 'future public health'.

The public health challenges of modernity

Many contemporary societies, and organizations and institutions within them, are beset by a series of seemingly disparate problems for which they are struggling to find solutions (Kelly 2006). The public health community, for example, is now familiar with the 'epidemics' of over-consumption such as obesity and problematic drug and alcohol use, which now plague not just the high-income societies of the West (Foresight Report 2007) but also middle- and low-income societies across the globe. Other significant public health issues include rising rates of mental distress and disorder (World Health Organization 2004; Layard 2006a), static or diminishing levels of individual and social well-being (Lane 2000; Offer 2006; Layard 2006b), and increasing health and social inequalities (Commission on Social Determinants of Health 2008; Wilkinson and Pickett 2009). Other emerging problems – which may at first glance appear unrelated to the above – include anthropogenic climate change (McMichael et al. 2006), peak oil (Roberts 2005), exponential population growth (Bartlett 1993), and ongoing global economic crises (Elliott and Atkinson 2008). All of these issues have profound implications for the health and well-being of present and future generations (Hanlon and Carlisle 2008). This book highlights the interconnectedness of such problems and argues that the public health community will need to draw on more 'synthetic' forms of knowledge in order to deepen and broaden its understanding of this vital point (Ehrlich 2000). In making the case for the future public health this book therefore draws on evidence and theory from multiple disciplines, including but not restricted to public health. Its key arguments are summarized in Box 1.1.

Box 1.1 Key arguments: modernity and public health

- All of human history has been characterized by change. A number of ages in our history can be identified, each with a distinctive outer world (social structure, economy, culture and physical environment) and inner world (belief systems, motivations, consciousness). Resource and population pressures have catalysed each change of age. To cope, our ancestors developed new outer worlds (technologies, social systems and cultures) and inner worlds (beliefs and values). The modern age followed this pattern: resource and population pressures catalyzed changes such as the agricultural and industrial revolutions. Over the following centuries our current outer and inner worlds emerged. This is the 'modern' world referred to throughout the book and briefly described below.

- The ability of modern people to understand, predict and control the natural world has largely been made possible through scientific and technological progress. The result of this 'understand-predict-control' phenomenon has been beneficial in many ways, bringing us economic growth and social development, better health and health care, and material prosperity. Four periods of great progress in public health can also be identified over the modern period (described in Chapters 2 and 3). However, many social commentators have observed that the values of Western society have changed in parallel with changes to our economy and our social structure. These changes have been associated with the abandonment of many traditional sources of meaning and purpose in life and the erosion of a way of life based on production. We have witnessed the emergence of a post-scarcity society and a culture which places a high value on individualism and materialism. Our economic system is now driven largely by consumption. These trends have produced a mindset or worldview quite different from that of our ancestors.

- Evidence is now accumulating that this mindset is producing adverse effects for public health (Carlisle and Hanlon 2007; Carlisle et al. 2009). Similarly, the methods which were successful in the early period of modernity, and led to profound improvements in public health, are now subject to diminishing returns. One manifestation of the problems of modernity can be seen in the rise of new 'epidemics' such as obesity, a range of addictive behaviours, loss of well-being, and rising rates of depression and anxiety. For these public health challenges the tools of modernity have proven largely unsuccessful. Wider indications of the perverse but unintended outcomes of the modern, consumption-driven way of life include anthropogenic climate change, global economic crises, the loss of many other species (with unpredictable effects), and the depletion of key resources such as oil, land available for agriculture, and fresh water. In short, much about the modern way of life has been shown to be unsustainable, so there are profound implications for the health of existing and future populations. The middle chapters of this book address such issues in greater detail.

- The final section of the book stresses that the global nature of the problems produced by 'modern' life means that all societies will face inevitable

(continued)

> change. Public health stands in need of a new approach if it is to be suc-
> cessful in this changed future. This does not mean advocating a return to
> a pre-modern past: much that is valuable about modernity will need to be
> preserved. And the public health community needs to identify the oppor-
> tunities to be found in the prospect of involuntary change, as well as the
> threats. To do this, it needs to re-orientate itself towards the future. The
> final section of the book presents a radical new model for the future public
> health and discusses the implications for its practitioners.

The remainder of this chapter outlines some of the above arguments, which are developed in greater detail in subsequent chapters.

Living in a changing world

There is evidence that human society is entering a period of change which is si-multaneously challenging, unsettling and inevitable (Harrison 1993; Bauman 2001). Yet on the positive side, humankind has obviously been in this type of situation before, as all human history has been characterized by change. With hindsight, a number of changes of age can be identified, each of which has had a distinctive outer world (social structure, economy, ecology and culture) and inner world (belief, motivation and consciousness). Resource and popula-tion pressures have catalyzed each change of age (Harrison 1993). To cope, our ancestors developed new outer worlds (technologies, social systems and cul-tures) and inner worlds (beliefs, values and consciousness). The modern age followed this pattern. Resource and population pressures catalyzed change and, over an extended period, our current outer and inner worlds emerged. Modernity is the term we are using to describe the period of time since the Enlightenment, one that has been characterized by a distinctive inner and outer world (Giddens 1991; Himmelfarb 2008).

The inner world of modernity has taught us to think of ourselves as com-plex biological machines that are the product of chance and time (Dawkins 1986). As 'modern' humans we understand ourselves as individuals, subject to biological competition (survival of the fittest) and social competition (the market). In 'modern' societies, the outer world is dominated by values of economism, individualism, materialism, and consumerism (terms explained below) (Featherstone 1991; Lury 2003; Ransome 2005; Slater 2007). We un-derstand the world both as a resource to be used and a complex machine that needs managing. We understand the task of organized society as satisfy-ing the inexorable, growing needs of the human population. Modernity also tends to have a narrow conception of science as the only legitimate source of truth, a view that is better called scientism (an ideology) rather than science (a method) (Hayek 1980; Sorell 1994). Yet we also know that the contemporary social, political, cultural and economic context in which we live has provided many benefits: for example, freedom of choice, individual rights, better health and social conditions and higher levels of material comfort for many. The problem is that these considerable gains have not been achieved without equally considerable costs. The sections below briefly describe these.

The costs of modernity for public health

One of the most significant of these costs, in terms of population health, appears to be a rise in rates of mental health problems and disorders (World Health Organization 2004; Layard 2006a); increases in a range of addictive behaviours (Alexander 2008); static or declining levels of well-being for individuals (Offer 2006; Lane 2000); and an accompanying rise in environmental problems (IPCC 2007; McCartney et al. 2008). Part of the argument underpinning this book draws on a body of public health research which suggests that the values of modern society are part of the many problems we face. Eckersley (2006), among others (Schwartz 2000; James 2007) suggests that mental health and well-being across all modern, Western-type societies are being damaged by particular aspects of contemporary culture. These cultural characteristics of modern society can be characterized as economism, materialism, individualism and consumerism.

- Economism is the tendency to view the world through the lens of economics, to regard a country as an economy rather than a society, and to believe that economic considerations and values are the most important ones.
- Materialism and consumerism represent the attempt to acquire meaning, happiness and fulfilment through the acquisition and the possession of material things. In the modern consumer society, material values rank higher than spiritual values. Non-material aspects of life may be squeezed out.
- Individualism has had many benefits but has also resulted in a social environment where the onus of success rests with individuals, as does responsibility for failure. As individuals we are subject to the tyranny of excessive choice and higher expectations of life, together with reduced social support and social control. This results in a sense of increased risk, uncertainty and insecurity.

The middle section of this book explores a number of examples that illustrate the links between such values and a series of challenges for public health. For now it is sufficient to note that the obesity epidemic arises from a kaleidoscope of influences found in the so-called obesogenic society (Foresight Report 2007), the genesis of which can be traced back to increasing economic growth allied to deep-seated social values of economism and consumerism. The UK's rise in alcohol related harm took off in the early 1990s when cost, availability and the drinking culture interacted to create the circumstances from which the alcohol harm epidemic emerged. Yet attempts to reverse these influences encounter arguments based on the values of economism and individualism. It seems likely that there are few prospects of making profound changes while the values of materialism, individualism, consumerism and economism hold sway. Policy can make some impact at the margins (and should seek to do so) but is unlikely to create radical change. Unless there is a reframing of our current perspective, ongoing rising trends in obesity, alcohol related harm and inequality appear inevitable. Policy initiatives may well be dedicated to reducing inequality, combating obesity and promoting sensible drinking – and many would claim this as evidence that modern values are egalitarian and pro-health – but policy and values both struggle in the face of the prevailing cultural ethos.

Exponential growth in a finite world

Three key dimensions of modern life are currently growing exponentially. All three are linked to the exponential expansion in human numbers and the escalating resource use of human societies. These linked phenomena are energy use, the economy, and the exploitation and depletion of the natural environment (Rifkin 2009). The problem with energy is captured by the phenomenon of 'peak oil'. In brief, this is when the availability of oil reaches a peak in production and the remaining resource becomes more expensive and more difficult to extract (Hubbert 1945). In the economy, the exponential growth of credit led to the credit crunch and the economic crises which engulfed various nations by the end of the first decade of the twenty-first century (Elliott and Atkinson 2008). The environment faces a variety of threats, the best known of which is irreversible anthropogenic climate change (McMichael et al. 2006; IPCC 2007). We explore such issues in greater depth in later chapters.

Human population is also in an exponential growth period, achieved because of two unique inputs of additional resources. The first was the colonization of the new world of North and South America – the 'New World' which appeared to provide for limitless human expansion – and the second was the discovery and exploitation of oil. Despite warnings from informed sources that we have 'overshot' the earth's natural resources and are now living on 'environmental credit', many societies across the globe are seeking to perpetuate this growth (Catton 1982; Brown 1996). We may already have passed the critical tipping points for climate change and oil production (Roberts 2005; IPCC 2007; Hanlon and McCartney 2008a, 2008b).

The point is that exponential growth cannot continue indefinitely within the constraints of a finite system (the planet Earth). The problem is that very few people understand either the dynamics of exponential growth or the certainty of in-built collapse in any finite system that pursues such growth patterns (Diamond 2006). So, one of the key arguments of this book is that change is inevitable. This analysis is not confined to public health practice but suggests that many other spheres of modern life are subject to similarly diminishing returns. As yet, however, there is little evidence that the majority of people are responding to the problems of modernity by developing positive change. It is possible to observe denial, resistance or, at best, passive adaptation. In short, it seems that contemporary societies are beset by a series of seemingly disparate problems for which we are all struggling to find solutions. The public health community, too, is facing a world for which it may be inadequately prepared and equipped. We have, in other words, what Homer-Dixon (2000) terms 'an ingenuity gap': that is, a gap between the problems we face and the availability of adequate solutions.

A role for public health

Understanding the inter-connected nature of the broader changes we now face is a massive and complex task which cannot be achieved from the perspective of any one body of knowledge. Many academic disciplines and other forms of knowledge contribute to this understanding. The public health community needs to know more about the nature of contemporary change (its origins, its current manifestation, its possible trajectory) in order to grasp the nature of the problems from its own perspective and for its own purposes. Public health as a discipline has a long tradition of drawing successfully on other forms of knowledge and insight beyond its own boundaries, so this is not an insurmountable challenge.

However, we also need to recognize that the health and well-being problems which confront us can no longer be addressed by our conventional forms of thinking, tools and approaches. This book argues that most of the solutions offered to the problems of modernity have little chance of working because they are rooted in the assumptions of modernity itself. As Einstein is often quoted as having said, 'we can't solve problems by using the same kind of thinking we used when we created them'. If we cannot predict what will happen next but can be sure that change is coming, a number of questions arise. How can we make the transition to a radically different future world – efficiently, safely and with minimum harm? Evidence and experience suggests that we will only make small *voluntary* changes for health and well-being benefits. However, if change is *inevitable* – if we are forced to change by larger, irresistible forces – then we have the opportunity to reframe the current assumptions and ethos of modern societies. We also have a real opportunity to reframe some of the debates that inform public health policy.

Public health as a discipline has a vital role in acting on some of the issues briefly outlined in this chapter, through its own scientific base, its ability to grasp and use the knowledge of other disciplines, and its capacity for advocacy and political courage. But in order to do so it must confront the need for a future orientation – taking action today to protect and promote health for tomorrow's people. Public health as a discipline should set its sight on creating and sustaining the conditions for health and well-being long into the future. An important role for the public health community lies in fostering a change in mindset or worldview in order to promote positive, transformational change and the transition to a healthier social and cultural environment. This book represents a step in that direction.

How the book is organized

Chapter 2 describes the history of public health in the UK in terms of four discernible periods or 'waves' of development and health improvement. It also describes the models of health and health improvement which are associated with the different periods. The broader point which underpins this chapter is that one can trace relationships between the waves and emerging ideas about society, health and well-being. Because the 'fourth wave' is still with us, Chapter 3 addresses the more recent history of the discipline and describes some of its distinctive movements, such as the increasing emphasis on a sound evidence base for public health intervention, and the important health promotion movement known as 'Health for All by the Year 2000'.

The chapters in Part 2 of the book describe some of the public health and wider social problems associated with the late modern period in which we now live. These include: the enduring and apparently intractable nature of inequalities in health (Chapter 4); the question of how modern society, and the particular set of cultural values that have developed over this period, affect our health and well-being (Chapter 5); the rise in various forms of addictive behaviours, and of mental distress (Chapter 6); the problems associated with global demographic change (Chapter 7); and the overarching challenge of sustainability (Chapter 8).

The final part of the book draws together the many themes and arguments of earlier chapters and highlights the various implications for three key public health constituents: those relatively new to the discipline, such as students and specialist trainees: established practitioners; and those in positions of leadership. Chapter 9 outlines a new conceptual framework for thinking about health, based on the re-integration of science, ethics and aesthetics, in both their current and emergent forms. This integrative framework for health is then used, in Chapter 10, to speculate on a more sustainable future for both public health and the National Health Service (NHS). Chapter 11 begins the task of envisioning the future public health practitioner and the kinds of support they will need.

References

Alexander, B.K. (2008) *The Globalisation of Addictions*. Oxford: Oxford University Press.

Bartlett, A. (1993) The arithmetic of growth: methods of calculation. *Population and Environment*, 14(4): 359–86.

Bauman, Z. (2001) *The Individualized Society*. Cambridge: Polity Press.

Brown, L.R. (1996) *State of the World 1996: A Worldwatch Institute Report on Progress Toward a Sustainable Society*. New York: W.W. Norton & Company.

Carlisle, S. and Hanlon, P. (2007) Well-being and consumer culture: a different kind of public health problem? *Health Promotion International*, 22(3): 261–8.

Carlisle, S., Henderson, G. and Hanlon, P. (2009) 'Wellbeing': a collateral casualty of modernity? *Social Science & Medicine*, 69: 1556–60.

Catton, W.R. (1982) *Overshoot: The Ecological Basis of Revolutionary Change*. Chicago: University of Illinois Press.

Commission on Social Determinants of Health (2008) *Closing the Gap in a Generation: Health Equity Through Action on the Social Determinants of Health*. Final Report of the Commission on Social Determinants of Health. Geneva: World Health Organization.

Dawkins, R. (1986) *The Blind Watchmaker: Why the Evidence of Evolution Reveals a World Without Design*. New York: W.W. Norton & Company.

Diamond, J. (2006) *Collapse: How Societies Choose to Fail or Survive*. London: Penguin.

Donaldson, L. and Scally, G. (2009) *Essential Public Health*. Milton Keynes: Radcliffe Publishing.

Eckersley, R. (2006) *Well and Good: Morality, Meaning and Happiness*. Melbourne: Text Publishing.

Ehrlich, P. (2000) *Human Natures: Genes, Cultures and the Human Prospect*. Washington, DC: Island Press.

Elliott, L. and Atkinson, D. (2008) *The Gods that Failed: How Blind Faith in Markets has Cost us our Future*. London: The Bodley Head.

Featherstone, M. (1991) *Consumer Culture and Postmodernism*. London: Sage.

Foresight Report (2007) *Tackling Obesities – Future Choices: Project Report*. London: Government Office for Science.

Giddens, A. (1991) *The Consequences of Modernity*. Stanford: Stanford University Press.

Graham, H. (2010) Where is the future in public health? *The Milbank Quarterly*, 88(2): 149–68.

Hanlon, P. and Carlisle, S. (2008) Do we face a third revolution in human history? If so, how will Public Health respond? *Journal of Public Health*, 30(4): 355–61.

Hanlon, P. and Carlisle, S. (2010) Re-orienting public health: rhetoric, challenges and possibilities for sustainability. *Critical Public Health*, 20(3): 299–309.

Hanlon, P., Carlisle, S., Lyon, A., Reilly, D. and Hannah, M. (2011) Making the case for a 'fifth wave' in Public Health. *Public Health*, 125(1): 30–6.

Hanlon, P. and McCartney, G. (2008a) Peak Oil: will it be public health's greatest challenge? *Public Health*, 122: 647–52.

Hanlon, P. and McCartney, G. (2008b) Climate change and rising energy costs: a threat but also an opportunity for a healthier future. *Public Health*, 122: 653–6.

Harrison, P. (1993) *The Third Revolution: Population, Environment and a Sustainable World*. London: Penguin Books.

Hayek, F.A. (1980) *The Counter-revolution of Science: Studies on the Abuse of Reason*. Indianapolis: Liberty Press.

Himmelfarb, G. (2008) *The Roads to Modernity: The British, French and American Enlightenments*. London: Vintage.

Homer-Dixon, T. (2000) *The Ingenuity Gap: Facing the Economic, Environmental, and Other Challenges of an Increasingly Complex and Unpredictable World*. London: Jonathan Cape.

Hubbert, M.K. (1945) Energy from fossil fuels. *Science*, 109: 103–9.

IPCC (Intergovernmental Panel on Climate Change) (2007) *Fourth Assessment Report*. New York: Cambridge University Press.

James O. (2007) *Affluenza: How to be Successful and Stay Sane*. London: Vermilion Books.

Kelly, E. (2006) *Powerful Times: Rising to the Challenge of our Uncertain World*. Upper Saddle River: Pearson Education.

Lane, R.E. (2000) *The Loss of Happiness in Market Democracies*. London: Yale University Press.

Layard, R. (2006a) *The Depression Report: A New Deal for Depression and Anxiety Disorders*. London: LSE Centre for Economic Performance.

Layard, R. (2006b) *Happiness: Lessons from a New Science*. Harmondsworth: Penguin Books Ltd.

Lury, C. (2003) *Consumer Culture*. Cambridge: Polity Press.

McCartney, G., Hanlon, P. and Romanes, F. (2008) Climate change and rising energy costs will change everything: a new mindset and action plan for 21st century public health. *Public Health*, 122: 658–63.

McDowell, W., Bonnell, C. and Davies, M. (2007) *Health Promotion Practice*. Maidenhead: Open University Press.

McMichael, A.J. (1999) Prisoners of the proximate: loosening the constraints on epidemiology in an age of change. *American Journal of Epidemiology*, 149(10): 887–97.

McMichael, A.J., Woodruff, R.E. and Hales, S. (2006) Climate change and human health: present and future risks. *Lancet*, 367: 859–69.

Naidoo, J. and Wills, J. (2000) *Health Promotion: Foundations for Practice*. London: Elsevier Ltd.

Offer, A. (2006) *The Challenge of Affluence: Self Control and Wellbeing in the United States and Britain Since 1950*. Oxford: Oxford University Press.

Orme, J., Powell, J., Taylor, P. and Grey, M. (2007) *Public Health in the 21st Century*. Buckingham: Open University Press.

Pencheon, D., Guest, C., Melzer, D. and Gray, M. (eds) (2001) *Oxford Handbook of Public Health Practice*. Oxford: Oxford University Press.

Pomerleau, J. and McKee, M. (2005) *Issues in Public Health*. Buckingham: Open University Press.

Ransome, P. (2005) *Work, Consumption and Culture: Affluence and Social Change in the 21st Century*. London: Sage.

Rifkin, J. (2009) *The Empathic Civilization: The Race to Global Consciousness in a World in Crisis*. Cambridge: Polity Press.

Roberts, B. (2005) *The End of Oil: The Decline of the Petroleum Economy and the Rise of a New World Energy Order*. London: Bloomsbury.

Schwartz, B. (2000) Self-determination: the tyranny of freedom. *American Psychologist*, 55: 79–88.

Slater, D. (2007) *Consumer Culture and Modernity*. Cambridge: Polity Press.

Sorell, T. (1994) *Scientism: Philosophy and the Infatuation with Science*. London: Routledge.

Wilkinson, R. and Pickett, K. (2009) *The Spirit Level: Why More Equal Societies Almost Always Do Better*. London: Allen Lane.

World Health Organization (2004) World mental health surveys. *Journal of the American Medical Association*, 291(21): 2581–90.

2 The development of public health in the UK

Introduction

This chapter describes how the UK has seen several phases of public health improvement since the Industrial Revolution, each of which can be linked to major shifts in the nature of society and the emergence of different threats to population health (Lyon 2003). These phases can be conceptualized as 'waves' of development. Each wave rises rapidly and maximum impact is experienced during this period (Hanlon et al. 2011). Inevitably, the wave reaches a peak then declines in intensity. Although a trough of public health activity continues from each wave, none exerts the same impact as when it first emerged. This is not an argument for a precise number of waves or to locate these with strict historical accuracy, but to highlight the fact that one can trace relationships between these waves and emerging ideas about society and health. The waves of health improvement can also be understood as cumulative and interactive. It is important to understand that overall health and social progress has been maintained by a new wave starting while an established wave is *still rising*. The first half of the chapter describes each wave in some detail but in brief their approximate dates and key characteristics are:

- first wave (approximately 1830–1900) – classical public health interventions; the growth of municipal power and influence;
- second wave (approximately 1890–1950) – scientific rationalism;
- third wave (approximately 1940–1980) – emergence of the post-war consensus; creation of the welfare state;
- fourth wave (approximately 1960–2000) – effective health care interventions; focus on risk factors/lifestyle.

The second half of the chapter describes the models of health and its determinants and the models of public health employed in each of the four waves. This illustrates how health models change according to context. This part of

Table 2.1 Four waves of public health improvement

First wave	Second wave	Third wave	Fourth wave
Approximately 1830–1900: Classical public health interventions, such as water and sanitation, etc.; concerns with civil and social order.	Approximately 1890–1950: Scientific rationalism provides breakthroughs in many fields – manufacturing, medicine, engineering, transport, and communications, etc.	Approximately 1940–1980: Emergence of the welfare state and the post-war consensus: the National Health Service, social security, social housing and universal education, etc.	Approximately 1960–2000: Effective health care interventions help to prolong life. Risk factors and lifestyle become of central concern to public health. Emergence of nascent concerns with social inequalities in health.

the chapter describes the impact of these different approaches on disease, life expectancy and broader health outcomes. It also describes the changing demography of the UK, as changes in population size and in its birth and death rates are important in enabling us to understand the broader social context that shapes public health. The chapter concludes by identifying some key public health successes of each period.

Four waves of public health improvement and intervention

The four waves, with approximate dates for their 'peak' of effectiveness and impact, are summarized in Table 2.1.

First wave of public health improvement (1830–1900)

In the UK, the first wave of public health efforts to improve population health lay in the broader context of responses to social disruption caused by the Industrial Revolution. In cities, overcrowding, lack of clean water or sanitation, poor nutrition and a dire built environment created the ideal milieu for many forms of infection. At the same time, recorded levels of alcohol consumption, crime and illegitimacy (to quote just three indices) were so high that they suggest real strains on psychological well-being and social ties (Fukuyama 1999). The public health challenges of this period were initially seen as moral

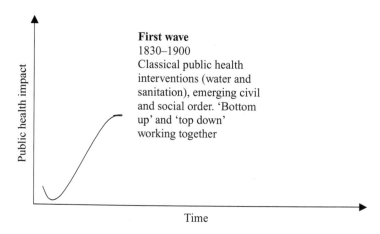

Figure 2.1 First wave of public health improvement.

problems associated with the perceived fecklessness of the poor (Wohl 1983) but this began to change following the work of early pioneers in the field of social medicine (Hamlin 1988; Hardy 2001) and Edwin Chadwick's landmark report (Chadwick 1842), which demonstrated the relationship between unsanitary living conditions and patterns of illness and disease.

'Great public works' can be traced to this period: the creation of reservoirs for major cities in the UK brought clean water to the urban population and the building of sewers was equally important. The growth of municipal power and influence also brought improvements in housing, living and working conditions and reductions in diseases before their causes were even discovered. Cooperative societies (Birchall 1997), modern police forces (Emsley 1999), health visitors (Buhler-Wilkinson 1987), orphanages (Peters 2000) and much else first emerged at this time (Wohl 1997). The new public health infrastructure therefore grew up around new governance structures: the development of municipal authorities, embryonic emergency services, and an emergent voluntary and charity sector (Hamlin 1988). The first wave can thus be characterized as the early appliance of science (when miasmic theories of disease were beginning to be seriously questioned if not discredited) and the development of rational social order, liberalism and the extension of the franchise (see Figure 2.1).

Second wave of public health improvement (1890–1950)

A second wave of public health was partly precipitated by the discovery of poor health in Boer War recruits. The second wave can be characterized by the rise of scientific rationalism, an approach also found in manufacturing,

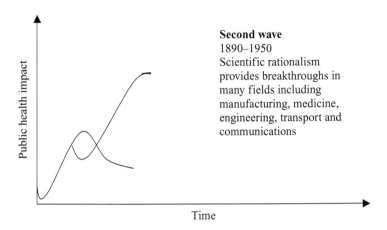

Second wave
1890–1950
Scientific rationalism
provides breakthroughs in
many fields including
manufacturing, medicine,
engineering, transport and
communications

Figure 2.2   Second wave of public health improvement.

medicine, engineering, transport, municipalism and the development of hospitals. This wave is thus based on the refinement of the appliance of science which had occurred in the intervening period. Scientific discovery suggested new approaches based, for example, on the shift from miasmic to germ-based theories of disease. The ideas informing all these changes can reasonably be traced to the rationalist philosophies of the Enlightenment period. The concept of the 'expert', a specialist in a particular and narrow field, is integral to how ideas unfolded in this context and gave rise to paternalist approaches to health care. The genesis of modern emergency services is also to be found in this period. During this period health became associated with the perception of the body as a machine – ideas which are still with us today. If reformers were key figures in the first wave, scientists like Koch and Pasteur were integral to the second (see Figure 2.2).

Third wave of public health improvement (1940–1980)

A third UK public health wave proved necessary following the Second World War as the five 'giants' identified by Beveridge (Want, Ignorance, Disease, Squalour and Idleness) had not been vanquished either by material progress or previous public health developments (Beveridge 1942). Intellectually, this wave was influenced by the materialist philosophies of radical social thinkers such as Hegel, Marx and Engels, who argued that material changes drive history and that society's institutions and modes of operation are shaped by the structure of class relations (Plamenatz 1992). Health was thus seen as the result of the conditions of everyday life. Such ideas can be seen in late nineteenth-century developments and throughout the twentieth century,

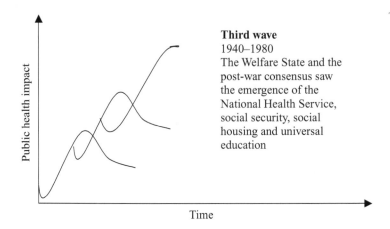

Figure 2.3 Third wave of public health improvement.

in the UK and elsewhere. Examples include the idea of universal education (Williams 2005), the welfare reforms of the UK 1908 Liberal Government, the Wheatley Housing Act of 1923, the post-Second World War settlement of the Attlee government which established the National Health Service, and the National Assistance Act, large-scale social housing and other welfare benefits. All of these had second wave roots. The key figures of the third wave were neither reformers nor scientists but politicians like Aneurin Bevan, the first UK Minister of Health (see Figure 2.3).

Fourth wave of public health improvement (1960–2000)

By the 1960s the results of the first three waves were clear: each had built upon its predecessor(s) and death rates continued to decline throughout most of the twentieth century (McKeown and Record 1962; McKeown and Brown 1995). At the core of the first three waves lay the idea that improved housing, education and health care, distributed fairly by a just government, would help cure society's ills. However, in the last decades of the twentieth century, organizations that delivered these public health measures faced increasingly complex challenges for which they were not designed and were not well suited. The UK became part of a rapid process of change that affected North America, Europe and parts of Asia. Many industrialized areas underwent a transition to become part of the post-industrial society predicted by sociologist Daniel Bell (Bell 1976). Service industries replaced manufacturing and a new knowledge economy emerged. Consumer choice exploded, fertility rates fell, divorce soared and out-of-marriage child bearing increased (Williams 2005). Trust and confidence in institutions declined while mutual ties between people became weaker and less permanent (Giddens 1991). Work and gender roles changed dramatically: greater control of fertility enabled women to seek activities beyond traditional child rearing and home making. The knowledge economy had less use for the physical strengths of men: in some communities a large cohort of younger men found themselves without a meaningful role at home or in work, and many lacked the education or social skills to remedy the situation. During this time, there were absolute increases in death rates in younger men from accidents, drugs and violence (Office of National Statistics 2001), and suicide (Platt 2000).

Medical interventions may have been responsible for much of the decline in mortality in the last quarter of the twentieth century but they provided few solutions to emergent social pathologies. In such a complex context the fourth wave became partly characterized by a concern for risky behaviours in relation to major disease patterns: issues such as diet, exercise, tobacco, alcohol and illegal drug consumption all loomed large in the conversation about what makes health (Rollnick 1999). Such risk concerns have also been extended to the area of mental health, where the emphasis is still mainly upon what makes individuals mentally ill and not on what supports mental well-being for the whole population. From about 1990 onwards, concerns about health also became influenced by systems thinking (Leischow and Milstein 2006). Policy interventions called for more integration between services and for them to relate their combined effects to health outcomes. The key figures of the fourth wave thus range from Sir Richard Doll, who first established the link between smoking and lung cancer, to Sir Michael Marmot, one of the key figures in the health inequalities research field. These and many others provided evidence for the public health response needed (Commission on Social Determinants of Health 2008) (see Figure 2.4).

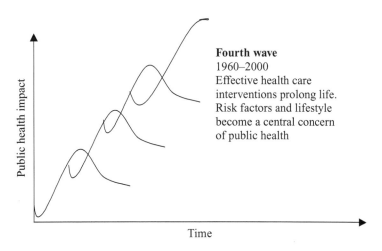

Figure 2.4 Fourth wave of public health improvement.

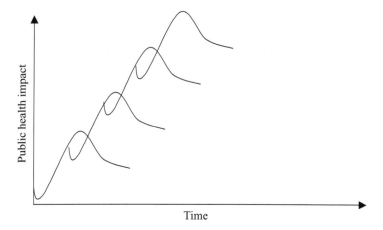

Figure 2.5 Four waves of public health improvement – cumulative and interactive.

Wave accumulation and interaction

As Figure 2.5 suggests, the effect of each wave is cumulative and interactive: much of what was developed through these four waves is still with us today. The developments of the first wave (for example, clean water and sewerage) remain vital to population health. The development of hospitals and associated professions which began in the second wave still continues and remains essential to the treatment of illness and important for actions to improve health. Increasingly, elements of the fourth wave (especially risk factors and the behaviour of individuals) have been integrated into these structures.

Emerging models: health, determinants of health, and health improvement

The term 'model' is used in the context of this discussion as a simplified representation of a more complex reality. All models of health and well-being are *constructed* in that their meanings are socially created and not natural phenomena. Such constructions are *contested* because not everyone agrees with any particular model or way of thinking. A range of quite different models and definitions of health have appeared over the years, largely driven by the interests and concerns of different disciplines and their practitioners. Public health practitioners need to be familiar with the main models and definitions of health and the determinants of health, as well as the various models of how health can best be improved. The theories we hold (our mental models, our conceptual and explanatory frameworks) are important because they drive our actions and underpin the systems of health care and intervention which we develop. Different *models of health* and different *models of the determinants of health* have implications for the ways in which we try to preserve and promote the former and how we understand the effects of the latter. The skilled public health practitioner needs a sophisticated understanding of all models in order to develop the wisdom to use the most appropriate model for particular circumstances. He or she also needs to be able to change from one model to another, as circumstances dictate. Different ideas about the nature of health and its determinants can be discerned within each of the four waves outlined above, as can different models of health improvement and health care. The following paragraphs briefly describe these, and the demographic characteristics of each period.

First wave conceptualizations of health (1830–1900)

The first wave of health improvement coincided with the early Industrial Revolution. The emergence of coal as a key energy source combined with the steam engine and other technological advances to profoundly change the way people lived, as the first industrial cities formed in the UK. However, the people who fled the land (because of famine or clearance), or were attracted to the city because of opportunity, brought with them the ideas and mindset of traditional rural people. As a large body of research from medical sociology and anthropology has shown, people from traditional rural areas tend to conceptualize 'disease' (a diagnosable pathological condition) in terms of 'illness' (the lived experience of being sick) (Helman 1994; Pool and Geissler 2005). Such traditional conceptualizations were beginning to be challenged at the time by emerging scientific ideas about disease.

First wave models of the determinants of health (1830–1900)

Many traditional communities have conceptualized the determinants of health in spiritual or supernatural terms. Prior to the modern era illness was often understood to result from such things as the ill-will of others (in the form of a curse or the 'evil eye') or from sinful behaviour (in the case of some religious communities). In both cases fate played a large part in most people's ideas about what caused illness to strike. Ideas of contagion had been appreciated for centuries but there was no understanding of the mechanism by which infection (the commonest cause of disease) was passed from those who were affected to those who were not. The concept of isolation had been understood since epidemics like the plague but thinking about hygiene was rudimentary at best. The theory of miasma (that disease resulted from the 'bad air' that hung over the emerging industrial cities) attracted considerable support until scientific insights provided a more convincing explanation (Bonita et al. 2006).

First wave model of public health (1830–1900)

In some respects, the first wave represents the golden age of public health. Health and social problems were so daunting and widespread that a massive and multifaceted response was needed. For example, the building of sewers in growing industrial cities like Liverpool, Manchester and Glasgow required political leadership, finance, engineering skills and considerable organizational talent. The earliest public health pioneers were often politicians, engineers, local leaders and business people, as well as health professionals. The first Chief Medical Officer in Britain (William Henry Duncan, 1805–1863) was appointed in Liverpool. He, like other early medical officers, was a clinician who learned his public health skills on the job. The first wave of public health was therefore not professionally led (at least in the first instance). It was also 'ecological' (in the sense that they recognized that it was the ecology of the emerging cities that was causing poor health and needed to change). Finally, the first wave can also be thought of as 'holistic' (in the sense that its practitioners confronted as many of the determinants of health as their understanding and resources permitted). From an altruistic perspective, their work was informed by a sense of social justice, as it was the poor who suffered the most illness and most lacked the resources to help themselves. However, those with the greatest wealth were also aware of the danger of contracting diseases from their poorer neighbours/neighbourhoods.

First wave model of health care (1830–1900)

During the first wave of public health development, health care was rudimentary at best. There were very few buildings or facilities and ideas of hygiene and asepsis developed slowly. Lister developed asepsis in 1865, Pasteur's germ theory emerged in 1862 and Florence Nightingale's notes on nursing were published in 1859. As medical technology was so rudimentary doctors relied much more on what we now recognize as the intrinsic capacity of the body to heal itself in many cases. Self-care and untrained mutual care, combined with lay knowledge (in areas such as midwifery, for example) was a common approach.

Demography of the first wave (1830–1900)

Pre-industrial Britain had been characterized by a balance between birth rates and death rates. Birth and death rates were very high and their approximate balance resulted in very slow population growth. Birth and fertility rates were high for many reasons. Children cost little to rear and were able to contribute to the family economy, while lack of family planning, religious beliefs and long tradition encouraged large families. Children were an insurance policy for parents whose only means of support might come from the continuation of the family farm or business or other support from their children as working adults. High infant mortality rates also meant that parents needed a large family to ensure some children would survive into their own old age. Death rates were high due to high levels of disease and poor or no public health or health care. Famine, drought and other natural disasters contributed, as did lack of clean water and sanitation, malnutrition and poor diet, and the existence of diseases such as tuberculosis. High death rates affected both the elderly and the young; most people did not reach a dependent retirement.

The relative demographic stability of pre-industrial Britain persisted for centuries but by the beginning of the first wave of health improvement an imbalance had gradually developed between death rates and birth rates. Death rates declined by the late nineteenth century because of agricultural and industrial development. This was the start of a now well understood process known as the demographic transition, and the UK was one of the first countries to experience this. The key observation of the second stage of the demographic transition is that death rates decrease rapidly but birth rates do not. This created the imbalance that led to a large increase in population at this time. In short, population explosions happen because of fewer deaths rather than more births. Another effect of this stage of the demographic transition is a change in the age structure of the population. In the pre-industrial phase, most deaths are concentrated in the first five to 10 years of life. But in the second stage of the demographic transition, more children survive. Consequently, the age structure of the population becomes increasingly youthful. This means that more of these children enter the reproductive cycle of their lives while still maintaining the high fertility rates of their parents. This causes the 'bottom' of the age pyramid to widen first, accelerating population growth.

Second wave conceptualizations of health (1890–1950)

The opening of the period of the second wave of health improvement coincided with the end of the nineteenth and the beginning of the twentieth century. This was a period of enormous optimism and great belief in the idea of progress. In this atmosphere, concepts of health were influenced by the scientific thinking of the day. The body was conceptualized as a complex machine made up of components (body systems and organs) that could be subject to malfunctions. The task of medicine was to understand the functioning of the body and correct malfunctions when they arose. Doctors began to specialize in specific body systems and particular diseases.

Reductionism began to dominate ideas of health and brought with it such success that it seemed to carry all before it. In this context, reductionism means an approach to understanding the nature of the body by reducing it to the interactions of its component parts (molecules, cells, tissues, organs,

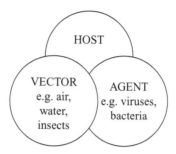

Figure 2.6   The agent-vector-host model.
Note: In this model the HOST is the potentially vulnerable human being. The AGENT is the causes of disease – mostly infections but also toxins and pollutants. The VECTOR is the means by which the agent of disease is carried to the person.

etc.). Some took reductionism still further and adopted the philosophical position that a human being is nothing but the sum of its parts, understandable through the accounts of biology, physiology and pathology. From such understandings emerged one of the most well known of all models of health: the 'medical model'. In this model, to be healthy is to be free from disease, which is diagnosable through physical examination for abnormal signs and laboratory tests that indicate abnormal physiology and biochemistry. Health services based on this model concentrate on diagnosing and treating ill health. It has proven highly successful in practice, not least because there are many occasions where attention to disease or other forms of physical damage is entirely appropriate.

Second wave models of the determinants of health (1890–1950)

During the second wave of health improvement a simple but often effective model of the determinants of health arose. Infectious diseases dominated and health was increasingly viewed as an absence of disease. Infections were understood by the new science of microbiology as deriving from a variety of pathological agents (viruses, bacteria, protozoa, etc.). To be transmitted, these agents need a vector: these included insects, water, air and other people. The person who contracted the infection was conceptualized as the host. This gave rise to the simple model illustrated in Figure 2.6.

Second wave model of public health (1890–1950)

The result of this thinking was that the host had to be protected from the agent, which could be achieved in a variety of ways. The agent could be destroyed (e.g. by disinfection); the vector could be controlled (e.g. by elimination of insect vectors); or, the host could be protected (e.g. by vaccination). Yet the first wave model of public health still remained relevant and effective. So the second wave saw a combination of progress in many fields (nutrition, sanitation, town planning, industrial safety, social reforms, wages, housing and so on) with the 'agent-vector-host' model to further improve health. Analysis of cause-specific death rates suggests that the first wave of public health improvements had maximum impact on water-borne infections while the second wave, mostly though improved living circumstances, eventually impacted upon air-borne infections. Importantly, greater understanding of diseases and prevention meant that public health began to see itself as a scientific discipline and a medical specialty rather than an agent of social reform. This crucial change altered the manner in which public health was pursued.

The second wave model of health care (1890–1950)

Towards the end of the second wave of health improvement, health care began to enter what we now understand as the era of scientific medicine. Nevertheless, there is a paradox here: scientific understandings of disease improved enormously during the second wave yet by 1950 very few truly effective drugs were available. Early antibiotics had only just emerged and the pharmacopoeia available in most hospitals was very limited. So medicine made little impact on population health at this time. Nonetheless, a trend had been established and by the third and fourth waves scientifically based medicine would be completely dominant.

Demography of the second wave (1890–1950)

During the second wave of health improvement the population of Britain moved towards stability as population growth levelled off through a decline in the birth rate. There are many reasons why the birth rate fell, including easier access to contraception and substantial increases in wages and general living standards. Greater urbanization had had two effects: it changed the traditional value placed upon fertility and raised the costs of rearing children. Perhaps most important of all, increases in the status and education of women meant that increasing female literacy and employment enabled women to have roles beyond childbearing and motherhood. Economically, a reduction in the value of children's work and a continued decline in childhood deaths meant that parents did not require the birth of large numbers of children to ensure their own comfortable old age.

Third wave conceptualizations of health (1940–1980)

The third wave of health improvement is inextricably linked with the rise of the Welfare State in the UK. In many respects, the disease model dominated this wave. When Beveridge created the NHS his focus was on the burden of disease and the need to treat it medically. At the same time other ideas were becoming important. For example, in 1977 psychiatrist George Engel proposed a 'bio-psycho-social' (BPS) model of health (Engel 1977). Engel argued that the medical model needed to take into account the patient, the social context in which s/he lived, and the role of the physician and health care system. The BPS model accepts the role of psychology and the social environment in influencing physical and mental health status. Other models considered the fundamental prerequisites for health. For example, the hierarchy of needs model developed by psychologist Abram Maslow can be understood as positing biological/physiological needs on the bottom rung on a 'ladder' leading to the highest human need, that of self-actualization.

Other models of health highlighted the multi-dimensional nature of health, and emphasized its positive dimensions. Most relevant for public health, the World Health Organization declared that health is a state of complete physical, mental and social well-being and not merely the absence of disease or infirmity (World Health Assembly 1948). This way of conceptualizing health represented an important advance in thinking and has inspired much research and policy work, yet even this is not without its weaknesses. For example, it has been pointed out that health is not best conceived as a state but as a fluctuating subjective and objective construct. It has also been suggested that this organization's definition of health is somewhat utopian and perhaps even unattainable. More recent thinking has attempted to move the focus away from thinking about health as an end in itself and towards thinking of health as 'a resource for living'. While this insight is useful it gives little concrete sense of the nature of health or well-being. It might also have been influenced by macroeconomic thinking about health. We might also argue that health, in the sense of being 'whole', is a fundamental quality of living things and thus an end in itself, rather than a means to an end; so it should not be considered in such a utilitarian manner.

Third wave models of the determinants of health (1940–1980)

Two different models of the determinants of health can be discerned over this period. Within the health service, the model shown in Figure 2.7 informed planning and practice. In this model, people get sick or hurt for a variety of unspecified reasons that do not need to concern policy makers. This process gives rise to 'needs' which the health service defines as 'the capacity to benefit

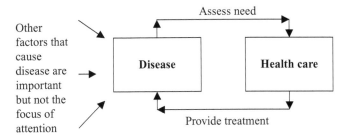

Figure 2.7 Model of the determinants of health employed by the NHS.

from health care'. Some people present with their health needs and others need to be identified (for example through screening). The health care system has a key role in interpreting and validating what the potential patient sees as a need. Of course, what is agreed to be a need depends on the state of medical knowledge and technology: advances in medicine discernibly increase 'needs'. Changing demographics also increase needs (a topic returned to in Chapter 7). The main characteristic of this model has been escalating needs and rising levels of health care provision. Adoption of this model with the resulting escalation of 'needs' and 'treatments' began during the third wave but became even more pronounced during the fourth wave (Evans et al. 1994).

However, this was not the model adopted more widely in the post-war Welfare State. Here, thinking was rather influenced by a structural and materialist analysis which understood that inadequate education, lack of social security, sub-standard housing, and poor health all related to and influenced each other. The policy objective was therefore to change material circumstances. For this reason, national and local government prioritized the building of hospitals, schools and council houses and the provision of social security and pensions. The pioneers of the Welfare State believed that a transformation in the material circumstances of the population, allied to the provision of high quality health care, would increase the health of the people of Britain to such an extent that the need for the NHS would diminish over time.

Third wave model of public health (1940–1980)

During the third wave, the role of the medical officers of health in large industrial cities across the UK became less important as the threat of infection declined and public health became an increasingly scientific endeavour orientated towards the understanding and control of chronic diseases like ischaemic heart disease, stroke, chronic obstructive pulmonary disease and cancers. This was the era in which epidemiologists like Sir Richard Doll established the health hazards of smoking and long term cohort studies were set up. This was also the era where the public health expert came to the fore and a wider range of specialties began to contribute to an increasingly professionalized public health (although public health specialists from a medical background still dominated the discipline in the UK).

Third wave model of health care (1940–1980)

Over this period the burden of disease changed rapidly in a process known as the epidemiological transition, which goes hand in hand with the demographic transition. Health care acquired a massive range of new investigative tools and therapeutic agents and an armamentarium of evaluation and research tools which, in time, would become formally known as 'evidence based medicine'. This was a period of great optimism that scientific and medical advances would cure an increasing range of illnesses.

Demography of the third wave (1940–1980)

Between the second and third waves of health improvement trends emerged that saw decreases in the birth rate and a continued decline in the death rate. The resulting changes in the age structure of the population included a reduction in the youth dependency ratio and, eventually, population ageing. In the UK, as in much of the industrialized world, a 'baby boom' generation was born in the period following the Second World War. These trends combined in a manner that was (at least initially) economically beneficial. The decline in youth dependency (as baby boomers entered the work force), despite the rise in old age dependency (as life expectancy increased), provided an opportunity for economic growth through an increase in the ratio of the working age to older populations.

By the end of the third wave (approximately 1980) the UK was in the stage of the demographic transition characterized by stability, with both low birth rates and low death rates. Birth rates were low because of the high cost of childrearing, the wide availability of contraception and rising opportunities in the workplace for women. This meant that most people were reluctant to bear large numbers of children. Death rates remained low due to improving health care and improving standards of living. Birth rates began to drop to below replacement level, leading to a shrinking population (although inward migration ensured that overall population numbers continued to grow). In this stage, the population age structure changed. Sufficient numbers of people lived beyond working age to create an enlarging cohort of dependent pensioners, supported by a proportionately smaller working population.

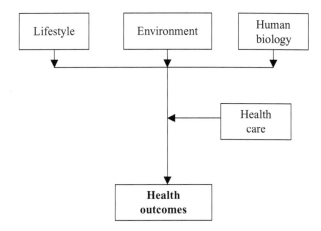

Figure 2.8 Lalonde's (1974) model of the determinants of health.

Fourth wave conceptualizations of health (1960–2000)

There is no single conceptualization of this stage. The fourth wave of health improvement is characterized by effective health care interventions and risk factor modification. Government policy and the NHS became focused on escalating levels of chronic disease. For example, ischaemic heart disease became a major concern during the 1970s: a disease model of health dominated the approach to diagnosis and treatment while a behavioural or 'lifestyle' discourse developed around the idea of prevention. A progressive public health analysis also developed, to explain the nature of health, the determinants of health, inequalities in health and much more.

Fourth wave models of the determinants of health (1960–2000)

In many ways the model illustrated in Figure 2.7, which saw disease and health care as the main focus, still predominated during the fourth wave. One of the earlier attempts to articulate a broader analysis at government level was the 'health fields' concept set out in the early 1970s by Mark Lalonde, Canadian Minister for Health (Lalonde 1974). His model (see Figure 2.8) proposed that the determinants of health could be categorized under four health 'fields': lifestyle, environment, human biology and health care. This model represented an advance in thinking but also led to a series of debates between two rival political camps. Those on the right of the political spectrum pointed to lifestyles as the key arena for action. They emphasized the need for individuals to take responsibility for their own health. The response of the political left was to emphasize the role of environment and call for improvements in, for example, housing, amenities and benefits.

Fourth wave model of public health (1960–2000)

Again, there is no single model to be found in this wave of public health improvement. During this period public health as a professional activity grew and diversified in the UK, becoming more multidisciplinary but also more professionalized. The dominant approach by government was risk factor modification with the intention of reducing the burden and cost of chronic disease. However, because this approach often placed the emphasis on individual behaviour change it attracted substantial critique. This model uses analytical epidemiology (primarily case control and cohort studies) to establish the 'risk factors' for a range of diseases and then employs education, treatment, social marketing and other instruments of government policy to change the level of these risk factors in the population.

This approach can be illustrated by exploring the relationship between systolic blood pressure (SBP) and stroke shown in Box 2.1.

Box 2.1 The relationship between systolic blood pressure and stroke

When the systolic blood pressure (SBP) of a large population of people is measured and charted, the shape of the curve is found to be a 'near normal' distribution. For most risk factors, the risk of disease increases with increasing exposure to the risk factor: so, the higher the blood pressure, the greater the risk of having a stroke. The risk is in fact curvilinear in shape so those with higher blood pressures experience escalating levels of risk. However, people at highest risk (i.e. highest SBP) form a substantial but not massive proportion of those who actually develop stroke. This is because they are relatively small in number compared to the very large numbers in the middle of the 'normal' distribution of blood pressure who have lower (but not no) risk. Very large numbers of people with lower but not insignificant risk generate more cases of stroke than the smaller number with highest blood pressures. As a consequence, most people who develop strokes do not have very high levels of blood pressure.

At an individual level, tackling those with the highest levels of the risk factors (that is, those with the highest blood pressures) makes sense, as they are at the highest risk of developing disease (stroke). However, this targeted or 'high risk' approach will not have a major impact on the disease in the population as a whole, as the proportion of people at high risk is relatively small. It is more effective in population health terms to target the whole population to reduce levels of the risk factor in everyone. This approach will have the effect of shifting the population distribution of the risk factor in a favourable direction, reducing risk of disease in both the high risk group and the general population.

Quite different preventive measures are required for the two approaches outlined. Treating genuinely high blood pressures with drugs is part of a high risk strategy while reducing the salt content of processed foods (and, therefore, the salt consumption of the whole population) is a good example of the whole population approach. The paradox is that more disease is prevented by lowering risk by a small amount in the whole population than by lowering risk by a large amount in the small proportion of people at high risk. During the fourth wave, public health strategists have applied the high risk and the whole population approaches to risk factors implicated in a wide spectrum of chronic disease with varying levels of success.

Fourth wave model of health care (1960–2000)

Health care has played an important role in the fourth wave of public health improvement. The model of health care became increasingly specialized and technical and the number of therapeutic agents of proven efficacy increased substantially from the 1960s onwards. Studies of avoidable mortality, inventories of health care interventions and analyses of age- and condition-specific trends in mortality have all suggested that health care interventions during the fourth wave have increased life expectancy and alleviated suffering at the population level. These analyses suggest that as populations become more affluent and healthier, the relative contribution of health care to improvements in death rates increases.

Demography of the fourth wave (1960–2000)

The risk factor and health care strategies described above impact most on older age groups: that is, they improve life expectancy by helping older people with chronic disease to live longer. The impact on the age of first morbidity has changed much less, so the length of time lived with chronic disease has increased. During the fourth wave, the UK moved into a new phase where birth rates have fallen below death rates. This stage is one that is now being experienced by countries like the UK that have undergone the economic transition to deindustrialization (i.e. the transition from manufacturing based industries into service and information based industries).

Public health successes 1830–2000

First wave public health successes (1830–1900)

One of the great successes of the first wave of public health was the control of water-borne infection in emerging industrial cities. This was achieved by providing clean water supplies and effective sewerage systems. Sewerage and clean water were strictly separated, purification technologies developed and systems of control and management established. This is a powerful example of the *understand–predict–control* approach which has typified the success stories of modernity. By this, we mean our growing capacity, since the Enlightenment, to understand much more about the natural world. The new sciences that emerged during the seventeenth and eighteenth centuries established cause and effect in the physical, chemical and biological spheres. For example, this allowed the behaviour of clouds to be understood at the level of molecules; physical forces to explain the movement of planets; the growth of plants to be made manifest by the study of cells; and the external characteristics displayed by animals to be explained in terms of genes. For public health, this mindset of understand, predict and control led to large and sustained growth in life expectancy. The control of water-borne infection was achieved by creating clean water supplies and effective sewerage systems. Practitioners of the time *understood* that sewerage carried diseases like cholera and dysentery. They *predicted* that separation of drinking water and sewerage would be protective and thus they succeeded in *controlling* infection. Yet we should remember that understanding of the science of water-borne infection remained quite limited at this time, and progress was made in the teeth of substantial opposition, and so required political as much as scientific skills.

When Dr John Snow, a physician and one of the fathers of epidemiology famously removed the handle from the Broad Street pump in London and thus helped to control the cholera epidemic, he did this on the basis of empirical epidemiological observations. (When charted on a map, cholera cases seemed to be concentrated among those who obtained their water from one particular street pump.) Yet the germ theory of disease and a detailed understanding of the bacterium responsible for cholera were not well advanced at that time. In short, early public health pioneers understood just enough to predict and control the problem and provide a solution. Detailed understanding came later, when chemist Louis Pasteur, surgeon Joseph Lister, and physician and public health pioneer Robert Koch developed, and gained acceptance for, germ theory.

Second wave public health successes (1890–1950)

The second wave of public health might be best thought of as the appliance of science, allied to continuing economic development. Our example of a public health success from this era is the development of vaccines. Perhaps the most spectacular success was with smallpox, a disease which was eradicated from the globe through vaccination in 1979. A wide range of infections can now be prevented with vaccination, of which the post-war programme against polio is another notable example. Arguably, vaccination is one of the most illustrative examples of modernity's ability to understand, predict and control.

Third wave public health successes (1940–1980)

The Welfare State in the UK is a prime example of public health success in this era. The Welfare State is a thoroughly modern project in the sense that it is a rational plan. It was this whole package, together with further improvements in living standards, which brought the third wave of health improvements to the UK. The Welfare State has brought: treatment free at the point of use to the whole population; social security; pensions; social housing; and much else. It is a collective endeavour that remains popular, despite problems, and a force for equity in an increasingly unequal society.

Fourth wave public health successes (1960–2000)

Declines in smoking prevalence in the UK represent a major achievement of the fourth wave in public health improvement and intervention. However, it took several decades from the emergence of scientific evidence about the harm caused by smoking until the first clear signs that smoking rates were beginning to decline. By the 1950s, Doll and Hill concluded from their studies that cigarette smoking is an important factor in the production of carcinoma of the lung (Doll and Hill 1950). Other early epidemiological studies showed harm from respiratory diseases, coronary heart disease and a variety of cancers (Doll 1983). Although this clear evidence of harm emerged in the 1950s, it took in the UK until the 1970s before smoking prevalence began to fall. Doctors assumed that warning people about the dangers of smoking would result in them giving up. In 1962 the Royal College of Physicians in the UK and the Surgeon General in the USA separately reported the dangers of smoking. Yet it took interventions in the following areas (working together) for several decades to really make a difference to smoking rates in the UK:

- price regulation;
- public education;
- social marketing;
- controls on product promotion, advertising and sponsorship;
- introduction of proven treatments;
- regulation of package design and labelling;
- point of sale regulation and legislation;
- pronouncements about tobacco and its industry;
- smoke free policies.

Smoking has thus declined because of a large number of synergistic interventions working together. It is impossible to isolate the impact of any one intervention without considering the interaction and impact of the others. While smoking bans have been a notable public health success they should be seen as part of a bigger picture of anti-tobacco campaigning and public health legislation. Multiple interventions (few of them supported by conclusive evidence of efficacy from trials at the time of introduction) were needed for this synergistic effect, and public health experts cannot be sure what aspects of which interventions were successful. In countries that have yet to employ this mixture of interventions, smoking rates are still rising. There are important lessons to be learned from this, expressed in the simple phrase 'it all matters'.

Summary

The four waves of UK public health improvement described in the first half of this chapter saw the evolution of a range of models of health, models of the determinants of health, models of public health, and models of health care. These varied models have been used by governments and the mainstream of professionals in the UK over the periods of the four waves. Over the whole period the population has changed from one with high birth and death rates and low life expectancy but rapid growth, to one with low birth and death rates, high life expectancy but high levels of later life morbidity and growing dependency ratios. The chapter has sought to illustrate how we can trace relationships between the four discernible waves of public health improvement, and emerging ideas about society, health and well-being. It shows how public health has been able to respond to changing patterns of disease and illness and ideas about these, to changes in political thinking and the structure of society (Szreter 1997), and to changes in its population size and age profile. The next chapter continues this theme in its consideration of public health today.

References

Bell, D. (1976) *The Coming of Post-Industrial Society: A Venture in Social Forecasting*. New York: Basic Books.

Beveridge, W. (1942) *Social Insurance and Allied Services* (Beveridge Report) (CMD 6404). London: HMSO.

Birchall, J. (1997) *The International Co-operative Movement*. Manchester: Manchester University Press.

Bonita, R., Beaglehole, R. and Kjellstrom, T. (2006) *Basic Epidemiology*. Geneva: World Health Organisation.

Buhler-Wilkerson, K. (1987) Left carrying the bag: experiments in visiting nursing, 1877–1909. *Nursing Research*, 36(1): 42–7.

Chadwick, E. (1842) *The Sanitary Conditions of the Labouring Population of Great Britain*. London: Poor Law Commission.

Commission on Social Determinants of Health (2008) *Closing the Gap in a Generation: Health Equity Through Action on the Social Determinants of Health*. Final Report of the Commission on Social Determinants of Health. Geneva: World Health Organization.

Doll, R. (1983) Prospects for prevention, *British Medical Journal*, 286: 445–53.

Doll, R. and Hill, A.B. (1950) Smoking and carcinoma of the lung, *British Medical Journal*, 2(4682): 739–48.

Emsley, C. (1999) The origins of the modern police. *History Today*, 49(4): 8–14.

Engel, G.L. (1977) The need for a new medical model: a challenge for biomedicine. *Science*, 196(4286): 129–36.

Evans, R.G., Barer, M.L. and Marmor, T.R. (eds) (1994) *Why are Some People Healthy and Others Not? The Determinants of Health of Populations*. New York: Aldine de Gruyter.

Fukuyama, F. (1999) *The Great Disruption: Human Nature and the Reconstitution of Social Order*. New York: Free Press.

Giddens, A. (1991) *The Consequences of Modernity*. Stanford: Stanford University Press.

Hamlin, C. (1988) *Public Health and Social Justice in the Age of Chadwick. Britain, 1800–1854*. Cambridge: Cambridge University Press.

Hanlon, P., Carlisle, S., Lyon, A., Reilly, D. and Hannah, M. (2011) Making the case for a 'fifth wave' in Public Health. *Public Health*, 125(1): 30–6.

Hardy, A. (2001) *Health and Medicine in Britain Since 1860*. London: Palgrave.

Helman, C. (1994) *Culture, Health and Illness: An Introduction for Health Professionals*. London: Butterworth-Heinemann.

Lalonde, M. (1974) *A New Perspective on the Health of Canadians. A Working Document*. Ottawa: Government of Canada.

Leischow, S.J. and Milstein, B. (2006) Systems thinking and modeling for public health practice. *American Journal of Public Health*, 96(3): 403–5.

Lyon, A. (2003) *The Fifth Wave*. Edinburgh: Scottish Council Foundation.

McKeown, T. and Record, R.G. (1962) Reasons for the decline of mortality in England and Wales during the nineteenth century. *Population Studies*, 16: 94–122.

McKeown, T. and Brown, R.G. (1995) Medical evidence related to English population changes in the eighteenth century. *Population Studies*, 9: 119–41.

Office of National Statistics (2001) *Social Focus on Men*. Basingstoke: Palgrave.

Peters, L. (2000) *Orphan Texts: Victorian Orphans, Culture and Empire*. Manchester: Manchester University Press.

Plamenatz, J. (1992) *Man and Society: Political and Social Theories from Machiavelli to Marx: Hegel, Marx and Engels and the Idea of Progress*. London: Longman.

Platt, S. (2000) Suicide risk among adults in Scotland: examining the evidence, explaining the trends, and reviewing options for prevention. In: A. Morton and J. Francis (eds) *The Sorrows Of Young Men: Exploring their Increasing Risk of Suicide*. Occasional Paper No 45, CTPI. Edinburgh: University of Edinburgh.

Pool, R. and Geissler, W. (2005) *Medical Anthropology: Understanding Public Health*. Maidenhead: Open University Press.

Rollnick, S. (1999) *Health Behaviour Change: A Guide for Practitioners*. Edinburgh: Churchill Livingstone.

Szreter, S. (1997) Economic growth, disruption, deprivation, disease and death: on the importance of the politics of public health for development. *Population Development Review*, 23: 693–728.

Williams, B. (2005) *Victorian Britain*. London: Jarrold Publishing.

Wohl, A.S. (1997) *The Eternal Slum: Housing and Social Policy in Victorian London*. London: Arnold.

Wohl, A.S. (1983) *Endangered Lives: Public Health in Victorian Britain*. London: J.M. Dent.

World Health Assembly (1948) Preamble to the Constitution of the World Health Organization as adopted by the International Health Conference, New York. Geneva: World Health Organisation.

3 Public health today

Introduction

This chapter begins by briefly describing the character of public health today – how public health understands its role in modern society, its areas of expert practice and its characteristic activities. This introductory section is intentionally short as much more comprehensive introductions to the subject already exist (e.g. Pencheon et al. 2001; Bonita and Beaglehole 2004; Bailey et al. 2005; Pomerleau and McKee 2005; Orme et al. 2007; Donaldson and Scally 2009). Pursuing the theme of historical development in public health, the mid-section of the chapter provides a critical analysis of two significant but quite different aspects of public health thinking and practice which emerged in the second half of the twentieth century. These remain influential and form a key part of public health development: the first is known as the Health for All movement (World Health Organization 1981), and the second is the evidence-based public health movement. These two movements illustrate the intrinsically political context wherein public health thinking and practice takes place, and highlight some important tensions within the discipline itself. A critical analysis of the movements is presented, leading to the conclusion that both Health for All and the evidence-based public health movement remain firmly rooted in the fourth wave of public health development. They do not, therefore, constitute a fifth wave for public health. The chapter concludes with a brief summary of the value and limitations of the four waves for public health today.

Public health: purpose and practice

The Faculty of Public Health is the standard-setting body for specialists in public health in the United Kingdom. Formerly the Faculty of Community Medicine and then the Faculty of Public Health Medicine, today's Faculty of

Public Health was formed in 1972 by the three Royal Colleges of Physicians (London, Edinburgh and Glasgow).

The UK Faculty seeks to promote public health through:

- promoting the education of all public health practitioners;
- examining all public health practitioners;
- promoting the profession of public health;
- developing and advocating policies for improving public health.

The Faculty defines public health as the science and art of preventing disease, prolonging life and promoting health in defined populations through organized efforts of society. This definition illustrates what might be called the essence of public health, where the focus is on improving the health of populations by a variety of means (prevention, protection and promotion). The definition implies that health is influenced by a wide set of determinants and so needs to be addressed by collective and state action (the organized efforts of society). It also implies a balance between science and art, although quite what the art of public health might be is rarely clarified. The Faculty describes three overlapping domains in which public health specialists practise:

1   health improvement
2   health protection
3   improving services

1   **Health improvement** is concerned with improving the health outcomes of whole populations. As such, it seeks to reduce inequalities while at the same time shifting the mean and whole distribution of population health in a positive direction. Health improvement happens at the intersection of four dimensions:

   (i)   **Topics** are selected for focused action: for example, smoking, exercise or alcohol consumption (sometimes the topic is a disease like heart disease or cancer).
   (ii) A **target group** is identified: examples might include children, older people, unemployed people or those from a minority.
   (iii) A **setting** is identified: examples include schools, the workplace or a city centre.
   (iv) A **method** or methods are selected: for example, education, screening, social marketing, and so on.

   In this way a health improvement intervention is created by combining a topic, a target group, a setting and a method. So, for example, safety (a topic) might be improved by identifying children (a target group) in a deprived housing scheme (a setting) using peer education, traffic calming and improvements to play areas (three methods).

2   **Health protection** is concerned with the control of infection and protection from environmental hazards. So, for example, the vast amount of work conducted in an effort to contain the spread and then limit the potential harm to the population from swine flu in 2009/2010 was part of heath protection. Control of hospital infection, immunization programmes and protection of travellers are other examples. Health protection is also concerned with the safe use of chemicals and poisons, e.g. in the workplace. Radiation is another hazard and in both cases legislation and vigilant monitoring of levels plays a key part in the process. Readiness for all types of major incidents or emergencies (from flooding to an aircraft crash) also falls under health protection. A great deal of the work involves anticipating infection and environmental health hazards and undertaking formal assessments of risk and potential impact to help inform policy and planning.

3   **Improving services** comprises the application of public health skills to the efficient and effective use of health care and other relevant services. Thus, work on clinical effectiveness, improving cost effectiveness and ensuring rational and appropriate service planning contribute to this diverse body of work. Audit and evaluation is one of the important routine tools of professionals who specialize in this branch of public health.

These three components of public health can be expanded into the nine key activities shown in Box 3.1.

Box 3.1   Nine key public health activities

1   Surveillance and assessment of the population's health and well-being: for example, through ongoing needs assessments of local populations based on routinely collected data and new data collection.

2   Assessing the evidence of effectiveness of health and health care interventions, programmes and services. In the UK, the work of NICE (the National Institute for Health and Clinical Effectiveness) provides a good example of this.

3   Policy and strategy development and implementation: for example, public health analysis and advice to all levels of government. Specific examples

(continued)

> include tobacco and alcohol regulation, health protection, nutrition stan-
> dards, health service organization and much else.
>
> 4   Strategic leadership and collaborative working for health: provided by, for
>   example, the role of Directors of Public Health, who provide public health
>   inputs to both health services and local authorities.
>
> 5   Health improvement: for example, via locally based programmes to em-
>   power communities and confront the determinants of inequalities in health.
>
> 6   Health protection: this encompasses many forms of infection control in-
>   cluding vaccination, together with the assessment and control of potential
>   environmental hazards.
>
> 7   Health and social service quality: this is achieved through research, audit
>   and surveillance designed to assess service quality, locally and nationally.
>
> 8   Public health intelligence: for example, the work of public health observa-
>   tories in the UK.
>
> 9   Academic public health: university departments of public health employ
>   a wide range of qualitative and quantitative methods to promote under-
>   standing of the determinants of health, and develop/improve interventions
>   to improve health.

In the UK there is now a large, multidisciplinary workforce that pursues the broad range of activities described above.

Two contrasting approaches to public health intervention

Two very different approaches to public health developed over the course of the fourth wave of public health improvement (approximately1960–2000), which was described in Chapter 2. These approaches have been sufficiently sig-nificant in the history of our discipline to be called 'movements': the 'Health for All' movement (World Health Organization 1981) and the evidence-based public health movement (Killoran and Kelly 2010). Although both belong to the fourth wave they also draw on earlier waves. To oversimplify somewhat, the Health for All movement has drawn on the *ideas* of the four waves, while the evidence-based public health movement has (unsurprisingly) drawn on *assessments of the evidence* they provide. The relationships of these two move-ments to the four waves of public health are illustrated in Figure 3.1.

The 'Health for All' movement

The history of health improvement differs across countries. For example, many countries in Africa achieved independence from colonial rule during

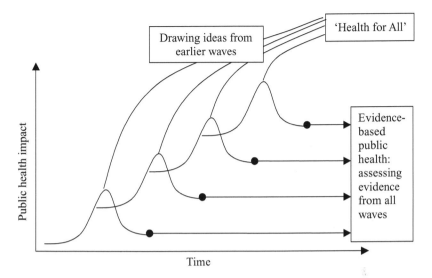

Figure 3.1   Relationship between the four waves, Health for All and evidence-based public health.

the 1960s and 1970s. These countries had previously operated with a dual system whereby traditional healing practices existed side by side with a colonial medical service. Independence created the expectation that the new governments would provide a high standard of health care, education and other services for their people. In response, teaching hospitals, medical and nursing schools were established, with support from donors. However, these were concentrated in urban areas, thus depriving access to populations in the rural hinterlands. Awareness of these problems stimulated the introduction of a new model of care: primary health care.

An international conference on primary health care, held in the former Kazak Soviet Republic in 1978, led to the unanimous adoption of the Alma-Ata Declaration (World Health Assembly 1978). The Declaration identified and recognized primary health care as a strategy for achieving health for all. The concept of primary health care was used by the World Health Organization and UNICEF to generate basic health care services that were equitable, accessible and affordable. The goal was to address the health care needs of developing countries, with more emphasis on prevention along with the provision of appropriate curative services. In 1977 the Thirtieth World Health Assembly decided that the main social goal of governments and the World Health Organization in the coming decades should be the attainment, by all people of the world by the year 2000, of a level of health that would permit them to lead a socially and economically productive life. This goal is commonly known as *Health for All by the Year 2000* (World Health Organization 1981).

Developing countries in Africa like Botswana, Burkina Faso, Kenya, Tanzania, Namibia, the Democratic Republic of Congo and Ghana adopted the concept in their national development plans. A review of these countries by the World Health Organization, to examine the implementation of the primary health care policy agenda, indicated that considerable efforts in formulating and marketing the policy had been made (Hall and Taylor 2003). However, it also identified weak structures, inadequate attention to primary health care principles, inadequate resource allocation and inadequate political will as obstacles to the full implementation of the policy.

In 1986 the Ottawa Charter was introduced in Ontario, Canada (World Health Organization 1986). This Charter advocated a series of health promotion principles as contributory tools for achieving the goals of Health for All. The Charter focused on five action areas:

1   build healthy public policy;
2   create supportive environments;
3   strengthen community actions;
4   develop personal skills;
5   reorient health services towards primary care.

It called on the World Health Organization and other international organizations to advocate the acceptance and implementation of health promotion strategies and to support countries to set up health promotion strategies and programmes. The Ottawa Charter eventually led to the Jakarta Declaration on Health Promotion (World Health Organization 1997), a further visionary statement of the development of health promotion. However, at the time of the Ottawa Charter (the latter end of the 1980s) conservative (or neo-liberal) political forces in North America and Europe were imposing structural readjustment programmes on developing countries and encouraging market-led mechanisms for health care at home. The authors of this book know that the principles of the Ottawa Charter were found deeply appealing by many working in public health, but we are also aware that many believe these principles were resisted to some extent by the UK and other governments and therefore never fully implemented. The response of the World Health Organization was to bypass UK and other national governments and form links with city administrations, many of whom were more sympathetic to the Ottawa Charter vision. This is how the 'Healthy Cities' movement was formed (Ashton 1991; De Leeuw 2001). An influential public health text of the time (Ashton and Seymour 1998) articulated health for all principles in a UK context, and the health promotion movement expanded considerably (Naidoo and Wills 2000; McDowell et al. 2007).

Limitations of 'Health for All'

Although the 'Health for All' philosophy and the principles enshrined in the Ottawa Charter remain relevant and important, history tells us they are not enough. In the UK, for all the impact of Healthy Cities and health promotion, the government and certain elements within the public health establishment resisted these ideas as lacking sufficient evidence or as politically impractical (personal communication). Even the World Health Organization in Europe shifted its emphasis over time (World Health Organization 1995). Those who had been involved in population-based risk factor programmes and public health interventions targeting chronic disease gradually gained influence and argued successfully the merits of focusing on these issues, at the expense of inequities in health and the wider determinants of health. Although the Health for All movement was motivated by an ethical imperative to reduce global inequalities and provide health care (and other basic ingredients of life as a stepping stone to this larger goal), the broader public health debate came to be dominated by concerns about disease risk factors, the role of evidence, and the perceived achievability of public health goals.

While it is widely accepted that population health is a product of the complex interaction of multiple determinants, there is still debate about the relative contribution that different determinants have made and will make to population health improvement. This debate has a practical edge when it comes to prioritizing interventions to improve population health. Much of the contribution to this debate reflects two widely held beliefs, attributable in part to the work of Thomas McKeown (1979). The first is that traditional style health services (as opposed to reformed, bottom up, primary health care services) have contributed little to the improvement in population health seen since the 1850s, and that the future role for health care in improving population health is limited. The second is that the NHS has remained a sickness service responding to illness rather than a health service improving population health. In response, some within the evidence-based public health movement have argued that, while these beliefs may have been true for the late nineteenth and early twentieth centuries, a number of recent studies warrant their reappraisal (Craig et al. 2006). And although the impact of health care on population health has still to be accurately quantified, this is also true of the other main determinants of health and of interventions to address them. In light of such uncertainty, two questions can be posed. First, why is there such a strong belief that health can be improved by tackling its non-health care determinants? Secondly, is this belief a useful guide to policy and if not, what (if anything) should be done about it?

The thrust of McKeown's arguments has gained strength from key reports, such as the Black Report (Black et al. 1980), the Ottawa Charter (World Health Organization 1986) and the Acheson Report (Acheson 1998), all of which drew upon a vast literature demonstrating strong associations between socio-economic status, environmental conditions and health. The persistence of these associations and the widening of socio-economic health inequality, alongside decades of massive and increasing expenditure and technological progress in health care, suggest the primacy of non-health care determinants of health, the limited scope to improve population health through increased availability and/or quality of health care, and the need to re-orient health policy and health services. A second factor is the high and rising incidence of iatrogenic mortality and morbidity. Although the aggregate effect on health of these two forces is difficult to measure, estimates suggest that over the past few decades, management of risk factors and better long term care of chronic conditions has had a positive overall effect on life expectancy and the quality of life. It could be argued that the 'Health for All' movement in the UK never fully acknowledged this evidence.

Elsewhere, resource-poor countries were forced to reduce their expenditure on health care due to high debts between 1980 and 1990. As a result, international donors like the World Bank introduced health sector reforms in the 1990s, as part of the economic structural adjustment programme in those countries. The World Bank made health sector reforms conditional for countries wishing to qualify for debt relief and financial aid. The health sector reforms emphasized the involvement of the private sector in the provision of health services (which often meant eliminating or minimizing government services). The reforms also focused on the rationalization of services and the introduction of user charges. These reforms were not without some benefit but were criticized for being driven by economic and political ideology and the failure to explain how such policies could be implemented in resource-poor countries with absolute poverty. So the vision of 'Health for All' was not fully realized in the developing world either.

Evidenced-based public health

It is important in decision making, policy development, and the establishment of new programmes to improve public health, that these initiatives be supported by scientific evidence (Killoran and Kelly 2010). Evidence-based practice is based on evaluation research that highlights interventions that have been found to be effective. The evidence-based public health movement applies the tools of empirical science to the interventions which have arisen from earlier waves of health improvement, in order to establish their effectiveness and cost effectiveness. As such, it has much in common with evidence-based medicine and evidence-based policy making. Evidence-based public health has established a set of methodologies (primarily those used by epidemiology and health economics, although others are also included) and a hierarchy of evidence. For many, the most convincing evidence comes from meta-analysis of a wide range of well conducted randomized controlled trials. There can be little doubt about the value of good scientific evidence and methodological rigour, or that there are many medical and public health problems that are suited to the evidence-based approach (Killoran and Kelly 2010).

Yet the evidence-based movement as applied to public health has not been without its critics within that discipline. Concerns have been expressed about the narrowness of the methods that lead to acceptable evidence (Nutbeam 1998); the difficulty of designing effective trials of interventions that may eventually have the greatest effect on health (e.g. policy interventions; Fitzpatrick 2000); the bias towards more proximal determinants of health at the expense of wider determinants (McMichael 1999); and so on. The limitations of traditional scientific approaches in deciding what counts as 'evidence' in community intervention are emphasized by the King's Fund's report on 'finding out what works' in complex, community-based initiatives (Coote et al. 2004). The report makes it clear that a rigorous approach to evidence can be combined with community development and capacity building, but only where specific and relatively straightforward health risks are concerned. There are other, generally more complex, health risks for which there is far less – or no – evidence of what works (Coote et al. 2004).

The problem is that paying attention to 'rigorous' and 'robust' approaches in judging what counts as evidence, risks obscuring the theories, ideologies, values and principles that underpin any form of health intervention, although these strongly influence what gets accepted as valid evidence (Raphael 2000). Is health conceived as the absence of disease or as a resource for daily living? Does the intervention focus on the individual, the community or the social structure? Is it about changing lifestyles, or about helping people cope with social conditions, or about changing those conditions? These questions involve values positions that direct attention to differing forms of evidence. Interventions that focus on education are likely to strive for evidence of changes in individual knowledge and skills. Those which aim for social action and changes in social norms are likely to be driven by community development principles, while those that seek change in organization practice and policy are engaged in health advocacy (Nutbeam 1998). The philosophy, assumptions and principles on which research is based have implications for both methodology and methods, and therefore the evidence produced. The greatest limitation of evidence-based public health, however, appears to be its inability to cope with the complexity and interconnectedness of the health problems of the modern world. This argument is explored below.

Limitations of the evidence-based public health movement

Hospital acquired infections provide a particularly useful example of how orthodox evidence-based approaches struggle in the face of modern public health challenges. Box 3.2 provides background information on the nature of such infections.

Box 3.2 Hospital acquired infections (HAIs)

HAIs are infections that are neither present nor incubating when a patient enters a health care setting. They are contracted by virtue of being in the health care environment and/or being subjected to interventions and treatments in such a setting. Some infections are spread from person to person; some are derived from the patient's own normal bacterial flora, while others may be the result of environmental contamination. In the UK, one in ten hospital inpatients has a HAI at any one time and dealing with this is expensive. Part of the complexity of this problem lies with the development of antibiotic resistance.

Antibiotics have been used successfully since the 1960s to control, and in many instances overcome, bacterial infections. While antibiotics have proved useful in the treatment of infection, their use (perhaps even their overuse) has led to the emergence of highly resistant strains of bacteria like MRSA (Methicillin Resistant Staphylococcus Aureus). These drug resistant infections are commonest in hospitals where high levels of antibiotic usage allow organisms to evolve, and the close concentration of people with increased susceptibility to infection allows the organisms to spread. The very old, the very young, those undergoing invasive procedures and those with suppressed immune systems are particularly susceptible and, of course, these groups make up a large proportion of hospital patients at any one time.

Clostridium difficile (CD) is a specific example of a HAI. CD is a bacterium that lives harmlessly in the intestines of approximately 3 in every 100 healthy adults. For these healthy individuals, the number of CD bacteria is kept in check by the presence in the gut of other harmless bacteria. CD produces spores that are very hardy and resistant to high temperatures. These spores are passed out with faeces and can persist in the environment (for example, on clothes, bedding, etc.) for several months or even years. If the spores get onto food they develop into bacteria in the recipient and in this way transmission is maintained without that recipient necessarily being aware of it.

However, if the number of CD bacteria increases greatly in the gut, it can cause problems. If, for example, a patient who has harmless levels of CD is given antibiotics for another reason, that antibiotic may kill many of the harmless bacteria that are present in the intestine. CD bacteria are not killed by most commonly used antibiotics so are able to multiply. The severity of the infection and the illness that follows can vary greatly. More severe attacks produce pseudomembranous colitis where membrane-like patches develop on the inside lining of the colon. This can cause bloody diarrhoea, abdominal pain, fever and, at its most severe, death. Anyone who receives a course of antibiotics is at risk of developing a CD infection.

However, most severe cases occur in people who are in hospital, or who have recently been in hospital. This is because CD bacteria and spores are more likely to be found in hospitals: people in hospital are more likely to have been given antibiotics and have underlying conditions that make them more susceptible to infection. CD infection may be spread from one patient to another in hospital although strict hand hygiene and other control measures have reduced the incidence of this condition in recent years.

CD infection is also more common in older people: over 8 in 10 cases occur in people over the age of 65. This is partly because older people are more likely to be hospital patients than other age groups but also because they are most susceptible to clinical infection. A further possible link is with the use of acid-reducing drugs which impair the natural defences of the stomach against this infection. As a rule, the longer the stay in hospital and the older the patient, the greater the risk of developing CD infection.

The evidence-based public health approach to the challenge of hospital acquired infections is to treat them as we have historically treated most health problems: we try to understand, predict and control the problem, and provide appropriate solutions. So, strict personal hygiene such as washing hands can reduce the spread of Clostridium difficile (CD), Methicillin Resistant Staphylococcus Aureus (MRSA) and other infections. Good cleaning practices and strict hygiene measures in hospitals help to prevent contamination of equipment and personnel with bacteria and spores. We also know that monitoring the incidence of infection and responding quickly to rising rates of infection is important, and can identify potentially vulnerable patient groups and target our strategies towards them. Indeed, professional, public and political concerns about hospital acquired infections have been so great that, in recent years, increasingly elaborate strategies to control these have been developed, although real success has proved to be elusive.

The continued application of evidence-based protocols to limit the spread of infection will be beneficial to some extent, but will probably only have incremental and marginal impacts. The root cause of the problem lies in the modern, industrialized model of health care. In this model, health care seems to be conceptualized as a factory for churning out episodes of treatment. In this factory system, the patient is conceptualized as a complicated machine with a broken part that needs to be fixed as quickly as possible. As a consequence, a whole new vocabulary has developed which speaks of efficiency, patient throughput, length of stay, cost effectiveness, and much else that is actually derived from industrial and economic models. Consequently, the numbers of patients that pass through a hospital have increased markedly since the 1980s and the length of time spent in hospital has fallen dramatically. This puts staff and systems under pressure, as well as increasing the pool of infectious pathogens that might spread from one patient to another. There are fewer opportunities for thorough cleaning, less down-time for reflection and fewer opportunities for a slower but more humane model of care.

This is exacerbated by a focus on targets for waiting times and by hospitals being funded according to the levels of activity they achieve: hospitals are paid on the basis of the number of episodes of care they provide, which is different from the number of patients they treat. Also, as the safety of medical technology improves (for example, anaesthesia), older and frailer individuals who would previously have been excluded from certain treatments on the grounds of risk are now treated. One key ingredient of the problem is the widespread use of a broad spectrum of antibiotics not just for humans but in animal farming, with the result that bacterial strains emerge that are resistant to antibiotics.

It is clear that the problem of hospital acquired infection has arisen as a side effect of the system of medical care created in the modern period. Logically therefore, even more rigorous applications of the mindset that created this system are unlikely to generate a radical solution. Hospital acquired infections are an emergent property of the complex system of factory-style hospital care that has been developed, alongside unintended consequences of decisions made by politicians (for example, setting waiting time targets) and farmers (using antibiotics). Another layer of complexity (protocols, restricted antibiotic formularies, a new cadre of infection control staff, hand washing disciplines and so on) may help the system to adapt and mitigate the worst aspects of the problem but will not alter the circumstances that gave rise to the problem in the first place. In sum, hospital acquired infections are a good example of how the public health community faces a series of challenges that are not amenable to what we might call the 'mindset' of the first four waves. This example illustrates a key limitation of evidence-based public health, in that it seeks to modify and refine existing approaches, rather than think radically about the nature of the problem and its solutions.

Value and limitations: legacy of the four waves for contemporary public health

The argument that current public health approaches are not sufficient to deal with some pressing and emerging problems does not mean that there is little to value in those elements of the four waves that remain with us. Nor does it imply that there is little progressive contemporary thought which can guide us into the future. Neither of these is the case, as the four earlier waves of health improvement remain relevant for UK public health today, and for the future public health.

For example, the first wave of health improvement remains inspirational in that, without a cadre of professionals trained in public health, politicians, engineers, entrepreneurs, activists and many others came together to create order out of what must have seemed like chaos. The first wave concept of prerequisites for health has also been adopted by the World Health Organization, which has pointed out that achieving and maintaining health is almost impossible in the absence of such basics as food, water, shelter, safety and so on.

During the second wave of public health improvement, the 'understand, predict, control and provide' mindset brought its greatest benefits. Health improved because of rising prosperity and improvements in many fields and disciplines. The appliance of science has brought many benefits that will need to continue and be shared with others. For example, the World Health Organization's expanded programme of immunization has, over the past three decades, brought cold chain and vaccine technologies to almost all the world.

The National Health Service, the great achievement of the third wave of public health improvements, has brought many benefits to the UK population. Its philosophies of treatment given free to all at the point of delivery and the provision of care for all from the cradle to the grave have provided health care services for several generations. Less obviously, perhaps, but just as important, the NHS has functioned as a source of social solidarity in the face of the rapid rise of an increasingly individualized society (a topic covered in more depth in Part 2 of the book).

The fourth wave of health improvement has delivered a considerable amount of learning both from programmes targeted at risk factors, and from the successes achieved by chronic disease management. The emergence of the 'Health for All' movement and the accompanying focus on health promotion has given the public health community a long-term vision of greater social justice and the reduction of health inequity on a global scale.

Nevertheless, and despite such strengths, the argument made in this book is that neither past nor present approaches to public health will be sufficient to cope with the ingenuity gap emerging from the current change of age. This is a large claim that requires justification, in order to explain *why* current approaches – even the most progressive amongst them – will not suffice. For all their successes, there remain significant limitations to the insights provided by the first four waves in public health.

For example, the 'engineering' approach to public health pioneered in the first wave still underpins housing-led regeneration efforts in areas of deprivation and poor health. Yet decades of research (Thomson et al. 2006) in this area suggest that the health impacts of many regeneration projects are inconclusive at best: new housing estates bring their own social problems and do not necessarily resolve issues such as health inequalities between more and less disadvantaged areas (King's Fund 2001).

The remarkable scientific and technological legacy and successes of the second wave have nonetheless been accompanied by many vaccine 'scares' and widespread public suspicions around genetic modifications of plant and animal food sources.

The third wave saw the emergence of the Welfare State yet its institutions are now staggering under the burden of ever-increasing costs and have so far failed to resolve inequalities in health and social outcomes (Office of National Statistics 2005).

The fourth wave's successes have been accompanied by an increasing tendency to mass medicate the population (for example, through fluoridating tap water or adding folic acid to bread). Despite developments across the range of medical disciplines we have also seen the emergence of iatrogenic illnesses, such as hospital acquired infections. The fourth wave also appears to suffer from the over-application of the factory model developed by industry over the course of modernity, and promoted in the health system because of its apparent efficiency. Neither the increasing strength of the evidence base for public health intervention nor the greater focus on primary care and community health development provided by 'Health for All' has had sufficient impact on the widening health gap between rich and poor nations, and the health gap and social gradient of health within those nations. The movement struggled in the face of influential disciplinary concerns with disease risk factors and the desire to be evidence based, and broader economic and politically driven concerns about the perceived achievability of its goals. Conversely, evidence-based public health has sought to modify and refine existing approaches, rather than think radically about the nature of emerging problems and their solutions.

This critique suggests that continued or even more intensive application of the four existing waves of health intervention will not be adequate for the new public health problems we face. Part 2 of this book describes those problems in greater detail and highlights some important disciplinary blind spots that hinder us from successfully tackling the public health challenges of modernity.

References

Acheson, D. (1998) *Independent Inquiry into Inequalities in Health*. London: Stationery Office.

Ashton, J. (1991) *Healthy Cities*. Milton Keynes: Open University Press.

Ashton, J. and Seymour, H. (1998) *The New Public Health*. Buckingham: Open University Press.

Bailey, L., Vardulaki, K. Langham, J. and Chandramohan, D. (2005) *Introduction to Epidemiology: Understanding Public Health*. Maidenhead: Open University Press.

Black, N., Morris, J.N., Smith, C. and Townsend, P. (1980) *Inequalities in Health*. Harmondsworth: Penguin Books.

Bonita, R. and Beaglehole, R. (2004) *Public Health at the Crossroads: Achievements and Prospects*. Cambridge: Cambridge University Press.

Coote, A., Allen, J. and Woodhead, D. (2004) *Finding out What Works: Building Knowledge about Complex, Community-based Initiatives*. London: King's Fund Policy Paper, November.

Craig, N., Wright, B., Hanlon, P. and Galbraith, S. (2006) Does health care improve health? (Editorial). *Journal of Health Services Research and Policy*, 11(1): 1–2.

De Leeuw, E. (2001) Global and local (glocal) health: the WHO healthy cities programme. *Global Change and Human Health*, 20(1): 34–45.

Donaldson, L.J. and Scally, G. (2009) *Essential Public Health* (3rd edn). Oxford: Radcliffe Publishing.

Fitzpatrick, M. (2000) *The Tyranny of Health: Doctors and the Regulation of Lifestyle*. London: Routledge.

Hall, J.J. and Taylor, R. (2003) Health for all beyond 2000: the demise of the Alma Ata declaration and primary care in developing countries. *Medical Journal of Australia*, 178: 17–20.

Killoran, A. and Kelly, M. (2010) *Evidence-based Public Health: Effectiveness and Efficiency*. Oxford: Oxford University Press.

King's Fund (2001) *Regeneration and Health: A Selected Review of Research*. London: Nuffield Institute for Health.

McKeown, T. (1979) *The Role of Medicine: Dream, Mirage or Nemesis?* Oxford: Oxford University Press.

McDowell, W., Bonnell, C. and Davies, M. (2007) *Health Promotion Practice*. Maidenhead: Open University Press.

McMichael, A.J. (1999) Prisoners of the proximate: loosening the constraints on epidemiology in an age of change. *American Journal of Epidemiology*, 149(10): 887–97.

Naidoo, J. and Wills, J. (2000) *Health Promotion: Foundations for Practice*. London: Elsevier Ltd.

Nutbeam, D. (1998) Evaluating health promotion: progress, problems and solutions. *Health Promotion International*, 13(1): 37–44.

Office of National Statistics (2005) *Life Expectancy at Birth by Health and Local Authorities in the United Kingdom, 1991–1993 to 2002–2004*. London: ONS.

Orme, J., Powell, J., Taylor, P. and Grey, M. (2007) *Public Health in the 21st Century: New Perspectives on Policy, Participation and Practice*. Maidenhead: Open University Press.

Pencheon, D., Guest, C., Melzer, D. and Gray, M. (eds) (2001) *Oxford Handbook of Public Health Practice*. Oxford: Oxford University Press.

Pomerleau, J. and McKee, M. (2005) *Issues in Public Health: Understanding Public Health*. Buckingham: Open University Press.

Raphael, D. (2000) The question of evidence in health promotion. *Health Promotion International*, 15(4): 355–67.

Thomson, H., Atkinson, R., Petticrew, M. and Kearns, A. (2006) Do urban regeneration programmes improve public health and reduce health inequalities? A synthesis of the evidence from UK policy and practice (1980–2004). *Journal of Epidemiology and Community Health*, 60(2): 108–15.

World Health Assembly (1978) *Declaration of Alma-Ata*. Geneva: WHO.

World Health Organization (1981) *Global Strategy for Health for All by the Year 2000*. Geneva: WHO.

World Health Organization (1986) *Ottawa Charter for Health Promotion*. Geneva: WHO.

World Health Organization (1995) *Countrywide Integrated Noncommunicable Diseases Intervention (CINDI) Programme*. Copenhagen: WHO Regional Office for Europe.

World Health Organization (1997) *The Jakarta Declaration on Health Promotion in the 21st Century*. Geneva: WHO.

Part 2

Modern public health challenges

4 Inequalities in health: an enduring problem

Introduction

Health inequalities are widely acknowledged as a key focus for today's public health community, and no single book chapter can possibly do justice to the wealth of complex material available on this topic. Numerous and varied sources of information and analysis on the topic already exist (e.g. Bartley et al. 1998; Graham 2000; CSDH 2008; Wilkinson and Pickett 2009; Marmot Review 2010). The purpose of this chapter is not, therefore, to provide yet another summary of the mass of evidence readily available elsewhere. Rather it seeks to give an overview of some important strands of public health thinking on this deep-seated 'wicked' problem (Blackman et al. 2006) and to illustrate some of the problems with that thinking – problems that have only become really apparent in recent times. As with other chapters in this section of the book, this one makes connections between a challenging public health issue and other forms of knowledge (evidence and theory) that help shed new light on the problem and prompt new forms of thinking.

It is nevertheless important to begin with a very simple point, by understanding what constitutes an 'inequality' in health. In almost all biological and social measurements, variability can be detected and measured. So, for example, if we were to measure the heights of young people brought up in good social circumstances in a country like the Netherlands, differences in height would be found. If these young people were ranked in terms of height, there would be a gradient. This gradient is not an *inequality* but a *biological variation*. If, on the other hand, we examined the heights of children who had been subject to malnutrition in infancy and were stunted in their growth, the difference between their height and the heights of well nourished children would be considered to be an inequality. There is general agreement that health inequality has a number of different dimensions, relating to social position, gender, ethnicity and disabilities. Having said this, the term 'health inequality' is used most frequently to refer to the differential impact that arises from the influence of a range of socio-economic factors such as income, social class and education. These social/structural differences are 'inequalities in health' because they represent a *systematic unfairness* that arises from the way we have chosen to order our societies (Wilkinson 1996; Graham 2000; Jackson and Segal 2004). That is, we can say there are inequities in health as well as inequalities (Oliver 2001).

The first section below provides a brief description of the importance of a lifecourse perspective on health inequalities, as different health determinants are important at different stages in life. The following section outlines the links that have been made between socio-economic inequality, poverty and deprivation as all have relevance for our understanding of health inequalities. The historic and apparently intractable nature of health and social inequalities is highlighted, and the distinction between the social 'gap' and the social 'gradient' in health is briefly explained. Some landmark public health contributions to the debate are then summarized, and the contribution of widening income inequalities in modern society considered. The complexity of factors involved in the creation of health inequalities is illustrated using health data from two very different parts of Glasgow.

As the material briefly summarized in this chapter shows, the health gap between rich and poor countries and between more or less advantaged people within countries has persisted over time (Davey Smith et al. 1999; Wilkinson and Pickett 2009). This suggests that inequalities in health constitute a worsening public health challenge and one for which a new approach is needed. The final section of the chapter makes the argument that a still wider perspective on health inequalities is needed; one that looks at how and why people's capacity for change might differ across the social hierarchy, and the ways that more advantaged people can act (semi-unconsciously) to *maintain* inequality. The chapter ends by linking the issue of health inequalities to the emerging challenges of developing a sustainable society and points to an emergent flaw in some significant public health thinking.

A lifecourse perspective on health inequality

One way of thinking about the factors that determine health in a population is the phrase 'it all matters'. What this means is that health in populations emerges from a complex interplay between the physical environment, social environment, individual behaviour, genetic endowment and the provision of services interacting with economic and other influences. These factors combine over the human life-span to create or destroy health and are responsible for observed patterns of inequality (Graham 2002). Different determinants of health operate at different times in the lifecourse, as the examples in Box 4.1 demonstrate.

Box 4.1   A lifecourse perspective on health inequalities

Pre-birth maternal nutrition can play an important role. The Barker Hypothesis (Barker 1992) was developed through an elegant series of studies which demonstrated that babies subjected to certain influences in the uterus that made them light for length seemed to be 'programmed' to develop problems like hypertension and diabetes in later life. In somewhat over-simplified terms, poorer nutrition in the uterus causes the infant's developing biochemistry to select pathways that are orientated to an environment where food/calories are scarce (this is known as the 'thrifty phenotype'). However, these babies are born into a modern world where food is overly abundant so there is a mismatch between their programmed biochemistry, their growth needs, and the environment they actually inhabit. The end result is a higher risk of a range of chronic diseases in middle life.

   Other important pre-birth influences include exposure of the foetus to alcohol and tobacco. A child's development, particularly neurological and psychological development, in the uterus and in the early years of life is crucially influenced by alcohol, drug and tobacco use during pregnancy and can be compromised.

The early years are increasingly being seen as important to healthy development. Psychologist John Bowlby developed what is called 'attachment theory', which suggests that the early attachment of the child to a caring adult (usually the mother) is crucial to neurological and emotional development (Bowlby 1953). Failure of attachment can have far reaching effects on behaviours like violence and the development of emotional intelligence. Our understanding of early neurological development is progressing rapidly such that it is becoming clear that insecure circumstances during early childhood impact on neurological development in a manner that is detectable in scans and, while not irreversible, can often prove intractable.

   Of course, the uterine environment and the level of support in the early years is a function of much wider determinants of health. Economic resources available to the family, levels of support and companionship, housing quality, normative behaviours, the person's inner life and a host of other factors interact to create these outcomes. Nonetheless, the point is that forces that give rise to inequalities in health later in life begin very early.

Childhood is a time when inequalities in health outcomes are relatively equal compared to later in the life course. However, habits of thought and behaviour are being established that will be very important as life progresses. The child learns empathy – the ability to put herself in the place and mind of another. This is a key skill and children who do not learn empathy are enormously disadvantaged. Childhood also seems to influence the development of locus of control, sense of coherence, level of self-esteem and other psychological markers that

(continued)

will influence health-related behaviours in later life. Diet in childhood influences weight gain and the risk of obesity as well as establishing lifelong tastes and habits. We are only beginning to understand how the regulation of the inflammatory system in the early years and childhood play a part in the risk of heart disease in later life. And so it goes on: a massive list of subjective and objective influences in childhood which are all socially patterned – that is to say, influenced by the social and economic circumstances of the family and mediated through norms, behaviours and the social and the physical environment of the child.

Adolescence is a time of exploration and experimentation. Much health-related behaviour is influenced by risk-taking patterns during this phase of development. Inequalities in health during adolescence are less marked than later in life but teenagers from poorer backgrounds are more likely to be exposed to parents and peers who are engaged in health damaging behaviours and are more likely to adopt these behaviours themselves. A further complication is the rise in a variety of mental health problems among all children and adolescents but with a strong bias to those from the most disadvantaged backgrounds.

The health of **working aged adults** is profoundly influenced by social position. The gradient in risk factors (smoking, poor diet, obesity, lack of exercise, etc.) is clear and can be best understood in terms of the outworking of influences from earlier in the lifecourse. This is compounded by a clear relationship between chronic stress and position in the social hierarchy (less status and income are associated with more stress). Poorer neighbourhoods have less good physical environments, more problems like antisocial behaviour, and these communities usually have less (bridging) social capital. The result is that there is a clear social gradient in all chronic diseases which has an impact on economic performance which feeds further into lower social status.

Late middle life sees the emergence of chronic disease and the need to develop and/or maintain functional capacity in the face of continuing disease. Evidence suggests that health in adulthood is the outcome of *socially* patterned processes acting across the entire lifecourse. Inequalities within and between populations are best understood in this type of complex and interactive framework. Graham has described this lifecourse-in-context framework as the joined-up science of health inequalities, one that brings together the concepts of cumulative exposure and pathways of disadvantage and locates these within changes in the socio-economic structure (Graham 2002). Poor economic circumstances are associated with an adverse position in many of the gradients which contribute to the final outcomes. However, there is probably no simple linear cause and effect but rather a complex system of causation from which poor health (mortality is just one of many manifestations) is an emergent quality.

Socio-economic inequality, poverty and deprivation

The concept of socio-economic inequality has long been linked to discussions of poverty and deprivation. Some key definitions of these concepts are illustrated in Box 4.2 as the distinctions made here are important in understanding the complexity and multilayered nature of inequality.

Box 4.2   Poverty and deprivation

The World Bank defines poverty as the circumstance when an individual must subsist on $2 per day or less (World Bank 2001). If this is 'poverty', can any citizen of a developed economy such as the United Kingdom truly be said to be in poverty? This tension is addressed by making the distinction between *absolute* poverty and *relative* poverty.

Absolute poverty is having insufficient income to cover basic biological needs. The United Nations declared, at the Copenhagen summit in the mid-1990s, that poverty is a condition characterized by severe deprivation of human needs, including food, safe drinking water, sanitation facilities, health, shelter, education and information (United Nations 1995).

Relative poverty is a less clear cut concept than absolute poverty. Townsend, a distinguished researcher in the field of poverty research, took the view that the necessities of life were more than the minimum amount of goods needed to sustain life. He concluded that the necessities of life are those goods that allow individuals to fulfil their role in society, participate in its relationships, and follow the customary behaviour which is expected of them by virtue of their membership in society (Townsend 1979). Operationally, relative poverty is defined in two ways. The first option is to consider income and an individual or family's position relative to the median income of the society in which they live. The alternative is to look at possessions and access to various amenities: here a shifting list of goods and services helps to define a notional 'poverty or breadline'.

Deprivation is a concept that gained prominence from Townsend's (1987) work. He points out that deprivation takes many different forms in every known society. People could be said to be deprived, he argued, if they lacked the types of diet, clothing, housing, household facilities and fuel and environmental, educational, working and social conditions, activities and facilities which are customary, or at least widely encouraged and approved, in the societies to which they belong (Townsend 1987). This combination of deficits is often known as **multiple deprivation.** In recent decades this concept has been extended to incorporate understandings of what happens to people experiencing such deprivation: they may become excluded from the conventional norms and behaviours of society. This is the concept of **social exclusion.**

We can understand from Box 4.2 that to be poor in the UK of the early twenty-first century is to experience relative, rather than absolute, forms of poverty, together with the potential for multiple forms of deprivation and social exclusion. Conversely, to be poor in the least developed countries of the world often means to experience absolute poverty (in addition to the other forms listed above, which may also be present). There are four elements that make the concept of deprivation relevant to public health understandings of health inequality. First, deprivation is multidimensional. Second, it is concerned with material and social (or relational) measurements. Third, it is *relative* – that is, it is based on socially accepted norms or standards which will differ from one society to the next and which probably change over time. Fourth, it focuses on individuals: it is people who are deprived and excluded, not areas. Nevertheless, it is the deprivation levels of small and larger geographical areas that are frequently measured and used in public health analyses. While this is useful, it must be remembered that not everyone who lives in any given area will share in the characteristics that define the area as a whole (McLoone 2001).

Public health research and political advocacy

The public health community has over many decades, and with markedly varying degrees of political encouragement and support, sought to explain inequalities in health and advocate action to tackle these. Responses to health inequalities have been debated and discussed, and various solutions proposed. Common themes thread their way through all the major UK reports on health inequalities. These are summarized in Box 4.3, which illustrates the steady accumulation of evidence, the broadening and deepening of public health understanding, and the persistence of the public health research community in keeping the issue on the political agenda.

Box 4.3 Key reports on UK health inequalities

The Black Report was commissioned by an outgoing Labour government but received by a new Conservative administration just after they came to power in 1979 (Black et al. 1980). The Black Report offers four explanations for the relationship between health and inequality:

1   **Artefact** – inequalities are not real but are an apparent effect that arises from the nature of the data used. This was investigated and discounted.
2   **Natural or social selection**, whereby ill or sick people drift down the social scale. This was investigated and considered to be a factor but quite a small factor in inequalities.

3   **Culture and behaviour** – health damaging behaviours and the cultures that cause them vary between social groups and cause adverse health outcomes.

4   **Social-structural explanations** – inequalities are caused by material and contextual conditions.

The report dismissed the first explanation above as lacking evidence, and attributed only a small proportion of inequality to social selection, the second explanation. The report's authors estimate that only between 10 per cent and 30 per cent of the socio-economic gradient may be explained by socio-economic differentials in health-related behaviour – the third explanation. They placed the greatest emphasis on the fourth, social-structural explanation for health inequalities and made a number of recommendations with a particular emphasis on child health. Although the receiving government ignored and even suppressed the report, it has since become not just an important historical source of public health evidence but an example of how the public health community acted to shared its insights widely among themselves and with others.

Some decades later, in the early years of a new Labour government, an independent inquiry into inequalities was established (Department of Health 1998). Led by Sir Donald Acheson, this report explicitly recognized the link between poverty and poor health and called for action across a wide range of agencies and organizations. Acheson argued that socio-economic inequalities in health reflect differential exposure, from before birth and across the lifespan, to risks associated with socio-economic position. He suggested that these differential exposures are also important in explaining health inequalities that exist by ethnicity and gender. Acheson's reference to the lifespan is underpinned by research that highlights how exposure to disadvantaged environments and to health damaging behaviour can have a cumulative effect over the life course, resulting in differential socio-economic inequalities linking directly to adult mortality and morbidity.

Fair Society, Healthy Lives, a further review of inequalities in health in England, was published in February 2010 (Marmot Review 2010). The report's origins lay in the UK government's desire to apply the findings of the World Health Organization's Commission on the Social Determinants of Health. The Marmot Review argued, with great clarity, that reducing health inequalities is a matter of fairness and social justice and that action on health inequalities requires action across *all* the social determinants of health. It suggested that to reduce the steepness of the social gradient in health, actions must be universal across society but with a scale and intensity that is proportionate to the level of disadvantage (proportionate universalism).

Marmot also argued that economic growth is not the most important measure of our country's success: the fair distribution of health, well-being and

(continued)

sustainability should all be seen as important social goals (Marmot Review 2010). From this perspective, reducing health inequalities requires action on early years, fair employment and good work for all who are able to, a healthy standard of living for all, the creation of supportive environments, and enabling and empowering approaches. Importantly, the review also linked action on inequalities with climate change.

Inequalities in health: an established and deep-seated social problem

In the Middle Ages, Britain's feudal society experienced profound inequalities in health that reflected the resources and opportunities of each rank or level of a highly structured and stratified society. With the rise of a market economy, social mobility increased and a different form of social hierarchy emerged. We are now living with the legacy of the long lasting, intractable and widening structural inequalities created by that market economy. For example, studies of parliamentary constituencies show that in broad terms the poorest and least healthy constituencies of the early 1900s occupy the same position today (Davey Smith et al. 2001). One hundred years ago the poor in Britain were dying from tuberculosis and other major infections. In the 1960s, inequalities in life expectancy were driven almost exclusively by ischaemic heart disease and other chronic diseases. Today, more of the differences between death rates in rich and poor are attributable to drugs, alcohol, violence and suicide in addition to the continuing impact of chronic disease (Leyland et al. 2007).

However, research has also shown that it is not simply the poorest people in society that experience less than optimal health, conventionally expressed as the 'health gap' between rich and poor (Davey Smith et al. 1999). There is also a *social gradient in health* across the whole population. This was illustrated by Marmot's now renowned study of civil servants (Marmot et al. 1991). The civil service has a strict hierarchy which determines salary, seniority and job type, and Marmot's work demonstrated a gradient of health outcomes across the whole hierarchy. Similarly, in the UK, each rank on the hierarchy of class, income, or education has, on average, better health than the rank below.

The widening gap in income inequalities

Figure 4.1 shows the trends in income inequality in the UK from 1975 to 2006 (Wilkinson and Pickett 2009). It shows how inequalities rose during the 1980s at the same time that Margaret Thatcher's Conservative government moved towards what are now called neo-liberal economic policies (Coburn 2000).

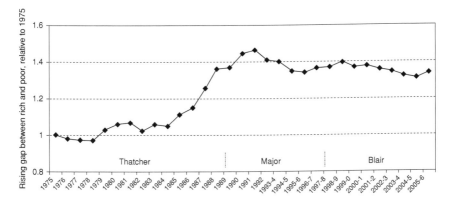

Figure 4.1 Trends in income inequality in the UK, 1979–2005/6.
Source: Wilkinson and Pickett (2009)

Subsequent administrations have largely maintained that status quo (Shaw et al. 2005).

As inequalities in income have increased in the UK, the gap in health outcomes between rich and poor has increased. Between the years of 1999 and 2007, for every 100 deaths which occurred before the age of 65 in the richest tenth of areas, 212 occurred in the poorest tenth (Wilkinson and Pickett 2009). This compared with 191 deaths in the poorest areas from 1921 to 1930 and 185 deaths from 1931 to 1939 (Wilkinson and Pickett 2009). In short, inequalities are at historically high levels in the UK. Similar neo-liberal economic policies were introduced in the USA with similar results: greater income inequality and greater health inequalities (Wilkinson and Pickett 2006). Neo-liberal governments have justified their economic policies on the basis that they would stimulate economic growth and that everyone would benefit: all boats are lifted by a rising tide. However, although Britain has become much wealthier in the period since 1979, income and health inequalities have increased too.

Apologists for the aggressive, neo-liberal form of capitalism argue that, while countries like America might be unfair, they are also successful and rich (Friedman 2002). This is a value judgement which is seldom presented as such. Moreover, even the more 'objective' dimensions of such arguments can be challenged. Large inequalities do not necessarily denote capitalist success but can just as well indicate imminent economic failure (Rajan 2010). For example, from every dollar of growth in income between 1976 and 2007 in the United States, 58 cents went to the top one per cent of households. The other 99 per cent of American families had to compete for the 42 cents remaining. The result was a country as unequal as it had been just before the Wall Street crash of 1929 – and with much the same results (Rajan 2010). Inequality levels among the most developed countries have also steadily increased since the mid-1980s both within and between countries. Thus, there seems to be an association with economic growth and increasing inequality both between and within developed countries during the period of economic growth from 1980 until the recession of 2008/9. Currently, there is insufficient evidence to suggest that greater inequality is an inevitable consequence of growth for poorer countries, as China and India are driving a reduction in inequality globally but increasing inequalities internally.

No simple solutions to a 'wicked problem'

Blackman and his co-authors suggest that health inequalities are a prime example of a 'wicked issue', by which they mean a complex problem which goes beyond the capacity of any single organization to understand and respond to (Blackman et al. 2006). Often there are no clear solutions to wicked problems and, indeed, they may never be completely solved but rather better managed as new knowledge about how best to tackle them becomes available. Moreover, there is often disagreement about the precise causes of the problem and the best way to tackle it. There may be an absence of evidence or what exists may be incomplete or contested, or both. Moreover, because of complex interdependencies, the effort to solve one aspect of a wicked problem may reveal or create other problems.

This conclusion is supported by data from community health profiles which demonstrated that the least healthy communities fare less well on a whole spectrum of indicators, not just health. Factors such as poor housing, unemployment, environmental degradation and inadequate or unavailable public services are mutually reinforcing, meaning that improvement in one small area is unlikely to bring about transformative improvement in others. It appears that a significant number of determinants of health would have to change for the health of a community to improve significantly. This is illustrated by the health indicators for two contrasting communities in Scotland: Newton Mearns (a wealthy suburb of Glasgow) and Dalmarnock (a relatively deprived inner city area). Figures 4.2 and 4.3 are drawn from a report which provides a detailed comparison of health outcomes and determinants of health in Glasgow (Hanlon et al. 2006). Each bar on the graphs represents that community's position on a specific indicator, such as death rates, hospital admissions, lifestyle factors, economic indicators, social markets and much else. So the indicators include both measures of health and measures of the determinants of health. Bars to the left indicate a position better than the Scottish average, and those to the right indicate a worse position.

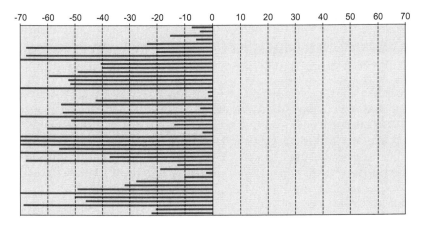

Figure 4.2 Newton Mearns.
Source: Hanlon et al. (2006)
Note: Current community health profiles for Scotland can be found at: http://scotpho.org.
uk/web/FILES/Profiles/2010

The comparison between the two contrasting areas clearly demonstrates the point that the least healthy communities have greater concentrations of multiple problems, not just fewer good health outcomes. Many (if not all) of these other factors will need to change before health outcomes significantly improve, and tackling each health condition or problem in isolation will not

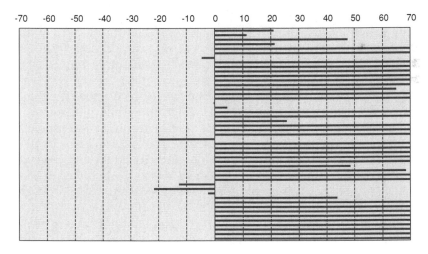

Figure 4.3 Dalmarnock.
Source: Hanlon et al. (2006)
Note: Current community health profiles for Scotland can be found at: http://scotpho.org.
uk/web/FILES/Profiles/2010

work. In terms of the four waves of public health improvement described in Chapter 2, Dalmarnock (the poorer area) already has the benefits of the first three waves. It has clean water and sanitation, access to preventive medicine and all the services of a modern Welfare State. In recent years it has also been targeted by the fourth wave of public health: programmes based on risk factors like smoking, diet and exercise. Yet these interventions are less effective in poorer areas because of all the other unfavourable social and economic factors that are at play. Modern medical interventions (such as statins for heart disease, high quality obstetric care and good cancer therapy) can benefit all populations and are available free through the National Health Service. Unfortunately, these interventions do not reverse inequalities because they fail to impact upon the underlying determinants of health.

Money: the bottom line?

Many people might acknowledge the complexity outlined above but would, nonetheless, want to bring discussions of what needs to be done back to issues of wealth and income. They might point to evidence that economically poor countries have very poor levels of health but modest improvements in their GNP brings about marked improvements in life expectancy. However, it is also the case that once a country becomes sufficiently wealthy to demonstrate reasonable levels of health, additional improvements in GNP are not associated with equivalent improvements in life expectancy. Indeed, the ranking of life expectancy among the developed countries of the world shows that the best predictor of life expectancy is the Gini coefficient (a measure of income inequality – see, for example, Wilkinson and Pickett 2009). What this demonstrates is that wealthy countries with fairer distributions of income within the population also have higher life expectancy for that population, compared to countries with the equivalent level of GDP but less even distribution of wealth (Wilkinson and Pickett 2009). The public health advocacy that flows from this is clear: improve the GDP of poorer countries and make the distribution of income in all countries as equal as possible.

The mechanism that links the Gini coefficient and life expectancy has been the subject of debate. The gradient of income could influence health through psycho-social effects: it is psychologically damaging for people, even the rich, to live in a society which is very unequal (Marmot 2004). Yet several economists have countered with the argument that additional wealth, if given to those who are already wealthy, has less value to them than the same amount of wealth given to those who are poorer (Lynch 2000). In short, spending money on the really poor is more efficient. What is absolutely clear is that, within a country, income is a strong predictor of health status: the rich are healthier on average and the gradient extends across the whole spectrum of wealth and income. Neither is there much debate about the fact that the gradient of wealth in a country has an impact on overall health status. However, it is still not clear whether income (or its lack) acts primarily through a direct material effect or whether it is a marker for other factors.

Widening our perspective

Contemporary public health advocates often argue that in more equal societies everyone benefits. From this perspective, enlightened self-interest should lead a country like the UK to move towards the distribution of income and other resources currently found in a country like Sweden. However, it must also be acknowledged that it is not possible for everyone to gain materially from greater equality. In material terms there will probably be winners and losers. It is perhaps more accurate to say that if a society moves to a more equal economic distribution, then cultural and behavioural changes will work though bio-psycho-social mechanisms as well as economic routes to favourably influence health, social and other outcomes.

Public health advocates – and others – can sometimes give the impression that if the UK had a more level distribution of wealth and income then that alone would lead to improved health. The Rowntree Foundation, for example, has published projected changes in mortality resulting from income redistribution, which gives the impression that benefits would flow from changing this single variable (Wheeler et al. 2005). This approach is part of a school of thought that frames health inequalities in neo-materialist terms. Neo-materialists argue that health outcomes result from the differential accumulation of exposures and experiences that have their sources in the material world (Lynch 2000). This perspective understands the world in mainly materialist terms.

A counterpoint to an overly materialistic analysis is provided by sociologist Pierre Bourdieu (Bourdieu 1984). Bourdieu's concept of the *habitus* plays a crucial role in accounting for the unthinking nature of most human action. The *habitus* can be crudely explained as the mental structure through which people deal with the social world. It can be thought of as a set of internalized (but largely unconscious) mental schemas through which the world is perceived and acted on. Bourdieu's work demonstrates the capacity of elite and powerful groups, rich in different forms of capital (i.e. economic, symbolic and cultural), to designate their own tastes as refined or distinguished while simultaneously defining those of people deficient in these forms of capital as vulgar or coarse. The stakes in these struggles are high, but the game does not take place on a level playing field. Since they have greater access to important forms of capital, dominant groups in society are able to bestow value on particular lifestyles which only they are in a position to possess. To be dominant in society is to possess the power to define and practise what that society values as legitimate forms of social distinction.

Simply addressing material manifestations of inequality will not address the complexity of the cultural issues around social inequalities in health highlighted by Bourdieu. If lifestyles can be seen as the product of the *habitus*, we can understand that people may have the *capacity* to change their lifestyles but will not necessarily be disposed or *motivated* to do so. Changes that do occur will tend to be in accordance with the underlying *habitus*. Put bluntly, eating 'healthily', taking physical exercise, learning to relax through meditation, and a whole range of other similar behaviours are unlikely to be part of the habitus or disposition of less advantaged groups. Conversely, groups high in cultural and educational capital are able to practise a key form of social distinction in contemporary society through extensive investments of this type. These insights suggest that, while economic and other social/structural factors are central, profound cultural and 'inner' change will also be needed (Carlisle et al. 2008).

Modern society: unequal, inequitable and unsustainable

It can be argued that inequalities are an emergent (albeit unintended) outcome of a complex adaptive system – the current model of advanced market capitalism. This is rarely acknowledged in any of the debates over discourses on and potential solutions to health inequalities. Some might even see such a statement as too political for public health professionals to make. Nevertheless, evidence is accumulating that the economic model practised within the developed world and increasingly pursued by the developing world is no longer sustainable and that change is inevitable. There is also evidence that economic growth produces diminishing returns for human well-being, once basic needs are met. This argument is explored in more depth in Chapter 5. For now, the reader is invited to consider Table 4.1, derived from work by the Global Footprint Network, which has calculated the number of planets needed to sustain the whole world, at the level of national consumption for various countries.

This requires some explanation. According to the New Economics Foundation (nef), forty years ago, if the whole world wanted to achieve UK levels of consumption, the planet Earth could just have supported the demand on its ecosystem (Simms et al. 2007). But consumption levels in the UK have risen steadily over time. Today, if everyone consumed as much as the average UK citizen, we would need more than three Earth-like planets to support their way of life (and that is before we allow for anticipated population growth – see Chapter 7). The UK's high consumption lifestyles are only possible because the rest of the world supports us with large supplies of their natural resources. The public health implications of this table are worrying.

Table 4.1 Number of planets needed to sustain the world at the level of national consumption

Country	Number of planets needed to sustain a national lifestyle
United States	5.3 planets
France	3.1 planets
United Kingdom	3.1 planets
Germany	2.5 planets
Japan	2.4 planets
China	0.9 planets
India	0.4 planets
Malawi	0.3 planets

For example, the redistributionist discourse identified above has a deep and enduring appeal for many in public health. It gives the impression that inequalities can be addressed by 'levelling up': that is, poorer people can be given material resources and power *without it changing the way of life of those who already have adequate (and more than adequate) resources and power.* Yet the global overshoot of the Earth's resources indicated by the New Economics Foundation and others, together with the threat of irreversible human-made climate change, renders this assumption implausible at best. What is now clear is that a conventional redistributionist strategy that seeks to level poorer nations and people up to the consumption levels of rich countries and people requires a level of resource that is simply not available. Global health and social inequalities cannot be solved by levelling up to the current economic activities of any of the countries in what we call the West (or the global North).

Yet, as political scientists and conflict analysts have noted, the globalized nature of communication has made many people in poorer societies aware of their own poverty and inequality, compared to the vastly greater material wealth possessed by those in affluent countries (Homer-Dixon 2006). This increases the likelihood of profound social unrest and revolt, even civil war, in many parts of the world (Homer-Dixon 2006). Equally, health and social inequalities within wealthy countries cannot be addressed by levelling up to the consumption patterns of the richest in that society. Structural-level action on health and social inequalities will certainly be needed, globally and nationally. However, it also seems likely that for health and social inequalities to diminish, a fundamental shift in some of the values which appear to dominate modern society will be needed. The next chapter explores the nature of those values and explains their problematic status for health and well-being at multiple levels: individual, social, and global.

References

Barker, D.J.P. (1992) *Foetal and Infant Origins of Adult Disease*. London: British Medical Journal Publishing Group.

Bartley, M., Blane, D. and Davey Smith, G. (eds) (1998) *The Sociology of Health Inequalities*. Oxford: Blackwell.

Black, N., Morris, J.N., Smith, C. and Townsend, P. (1980) *Inequalities in Health*. Harmondsworth: Penguin Books.

Blackman, T., Elliott, E., Greene, A. et al. (2006) Performance assessment and wicked problems: the case of health inequalities. *Public Policy and Administration*, 21(2): 66–80.

Bourdieu, P. (1984) *Distinction: A Social Critique of the Judgement of Taste*. London: Routledge.

Bowlby, J. (1953) *Child Care and the Growth of Love*. London: Penguin Books.

Carlisle, S., Hanlon, P. and Hannah, M. (2008) Status, taste and distinction in consumer culture: acknowledging the symbolic dimensions of inequality. *Public Health*, 122: 631–7.

Coburn, D. (2000) Income inequality, social cohesion and the health status of populations: the role of neo-liberalism. *Social Science and Medicine*, 51: 135–46.

CSDH (Commission on the Social Determinants of Health) (2008) *Closing the Gap in a Generation: Health Equity Through Action on the Social Determinants of Health*. Geneva: World Health Organization.

Davey Smith, G., Dorling, D., Gordon, D. and Shaw, M. (1999) The widening health gap: what are the solutions? *Critical Public Health*, 9(2): 151–70.

Davey Smith, G., Dorling, D. and Shaw, M. (eds) (2001) *Poverty, Inequality and Health in Britain 1800–2000: A Reader*. Bristol: Policy Press.

Department of Health (1998) *Independent Inquiry into Inequalities in Health: Report* (Chairman: Sir Donald Acheson). London: Stationery Office.

Friedman, M. (2002) *Capitalism and Freedom*, 40th Anniversary edition. Chicago: Chicago University Press.

Graham, H. (ed.) (2000) *Understanding Health Inequalities*. Buckingham: Open University Press.

Graham, H. (2002) Building an inter-disciplinary science of health inequalities: the example of lifecourse research. *Social Science and Medicine*, 55: 2005–16.

Hanlon, P., Walsh, D. and Whyte, B. (2006) *Let Glasgow Flourish*. Glasgow: Glasgow Centre for Population Health.

Homer-Dixon, T. (2006) *The Upside of Down: Catastrophe, Creativity and the Renewal of Civilisation*. London: Souvenir Press.

Jackson, B. and Segal, P. (2004) *Why Inequality Matters*. London: Catalyst.

Leyland, A.H., Dundas, R., McLoone, P. and Boddy, F.A. (2007) *Inequalities in Mortality in Scotland, 1981–2001*. Glasgow: MRC Social and Public Health Sciences Unit Occasional Paper no. 16.

Lynch, J.W. (2000) Income inequality and health: expanding the debate. *Social Science and Medicine*, 51: 1001–5.

McLoone, P. (2001) Targeting deprived areas within small areas in Scotland: population study. *British Medical Journal*, 323: 374–5.

Marmot, M.G., Davey Smith, G., Stansfeld, S. et al. (1991) Health inequalities among British civil servants: The Whitehall II study. *Lancet*, 337: 1387–93.

Marmot, M. (2004) *Status Syndrome: How your Social Standing Directly Affects your Health and Life Expectancy*. London: Bloomsbury Press.

Marmot Review (2010) *Fair Society, Healthy Lives. Strategic Review of Inequalities in Health in England Post-2010* (Chair: Sir Michael Marmot). London: University College London.

Oliver, A. (2001) *Why Care About Health Inequality?* London: Office of Health Economics.

Rajan, R.G. (2010) *Fault Lines: How Hidden Fractures Still Threaten the World Economy*. Princeton: Princeton University Press.

Shaw, M., Davey Smith, G. and Dorling, D. (2005) Health inequalities and New Labour: how the promises compare with real progress. *British Medical Journal*, 330: 1016–21.

Simms, A., Moran, D. and Chowler, P. (2007). *The UK Interdependence Report: How the World Sustains the Nation's Lifestyle and the Price it Pays*. London: new economics foundation.

Townsend, P. (1979) *Poverty in the UK*. Harmondsworth: Allen Lane.

Townsend, P. (1987) Deprivation. *Journal of Social Policy*, 16(1): 125–46.

United Nations (1995) *The Copenhagen Declaration and Programme of Action*. Copenhagen: United Nations.

Wheeler, B., Shaw, M., Mitchell, R. and Dorling, D. (2005) *The Relationship Between Poverty, Affluence and Area*. York: The Joseph Rowntree Foundation.

Wilkinson, R.G. (1996) *Unhealthy Societies: The Afflictions of Inequality*. London: Routledge.

Wilkinson, R.G. and Pickett, K.E. (2006) Income inequality and population health: a review and explanation of the evidence. *Social Science and Medicine*, 62: 1768–84.

Wilkinson, R. and Pickett, K. (2009) *The Spirit Level: Why More Equal Societies Almost Always Do Better*. London: Allen Lane.

World Bank (2001) *Annual Report, 2000–2001*. New York: Oxford University Press.

5 Public health, modern culture and well-being

Introduction

It is worth repeating here two of the arguments made in the first chapter of this book: that the world in which public health operates is changing faster than we can cope with, and that new public health challenges are emerging in an uncertain and unstable context, where existing models and approaches seem to produce diminishing returns (Hanlon and Carlisle 2010). Within affluent society, most people are now free from many former diseases and social constraints and many live lives of unprecedented material comfort. Equally, however, many people also seem not to be thriving in such a culture, in terms of their physical and mental health and well-being. There is, of course, the argument that the individualized, materialist, consumerist culture of some Western societies may be an inevitable companion to the spread of globalization, but is surely preferable to the misery of poverty and disease. This chapter turns to a deeper exploration of such modern-world issues but first there is the question of what modernity is.

The term 'modernity' is often applied to a period of time since the Enlightenment but it also implies a worldview that tends towards objectification, reductionism and materialism; a view of the world as lacking in any inherent meaning, design or purpose; and a view of the person as fundamentally separate, unique and alone (Himmelfarb 2008). In the modern, and newly globalized, world consumer choice has exploded and large rigid bureaucracies have become less effective at control through rules, regulations or coercion. The period from the mid-1960s to the present has also witnessed profound social change. Materialistic values now penetrate all aspects of life and a vast range of goods and services has become marketized and commodified (Gould and Gould 2001). Aspects of social disorder have risen while kinship as a social institution has accelerated its long decline; fertility rates have fallen, divorce has soared, and child-bearing outside marriage has increased (Fukuyama 1999). Trust and confidence in institutions has declined, as has trust in some 'experts' (Giddens 1991). Within local communities, mutual ties between people have tended to become weaker and less permanent.

Some of these changes can be seen – at least in part – as beneficial, in that certain forms of behaviour or choices in life are now less stigmatized, but their combined effects have been traumatic for some sections of society. In addition to the globalization of consumer culture and the loosening of social ties and traditions, there has been an explosion of innovation in technology worldwide which has led to what sociologists call the compression of time and space. In this globalized world, as the speed of transport and our power of communication increase, people paradoxically find less time for themselves and their families (Wilmott and Nelson 2005). Such are the profound changes of modernity, argues one of the foremost commentators on contemporary life, that many of us have no job for life, no partner for life, and no time for life (Pahl 1998). These are unprecedented conditions for a species evolved from a much more stable world.

As the whole world moves towards a single market in labour, all economies experience a widening of income, ranging from the highly paid (but time poor) knowledge workers down to unskilled workers in the manufacturing and service sectors, who may have to accept low wages or risk losing their jobs to international competition. Economies are placed under pressure to de-regulate to reduce costs and increase flexibility or risk losing investment to other parts of the world economy (Bauman 1998). The result, highlighted in Chapter 4, is greater inequalities in wealth within and between countries (CSDH 2008; Wilkinson and Pickett 2009; Marmot Review 2010): many parts of the world remain in absolute poverty. While age-specific rates of many chronic diseases are now declining, mental distress and disorder are increasing worldwide (World Health Organization 2001, 2005).

Health impacts of modernity

The health impacts of modernity for affluent societies are stark: we are overweight and overwhelmed. Analysis of these problems varies. Some have blamed a lack of adequate welfare provision and increasing poverty for the manifestation of social disruption, while others argue that current problems are caused by neo-liberal economic policies, too much wealth, and growing individualism and materialism. As Chapter 6 shows, rates of obesity and various forms of addictive behaviour, including alcohol and drug-related harm, are rising. In addition, we face the consequences of climate change (Intergovernmental Panel on Climate Change 1996, 2007), loss of biodiversity, financial crisis, and the decline of a key natural resource (oil) on which many economies now depend (Roberts 2005). Chapter 8 addresses such issues in more detail: the point is that such problems are not separate or discrete but interconnected and interdependent (Carlisle et al. 2009). To begin to explain this point, this chapter describes the relevance of a focus on well-being, for public health, and why our discipline needs a better understanding of how and why modern culture can influence this.

The relevance of well-being for public health

The concept of well-being has attracted sustained attention from many academic disciplines over the decades. This attention has also discernibly spilled over into the public and political domains. The popularity of well-being is clearly signalled by the thousands of readily available books on the topic (Nettle 2005). Well-being is now a regular theme in the UK newsprint and electronic news media and has considerable political appeal, with UK political leaders regularly referring to it in major speeches. Policies to promote well-being across the population may possess greater popular acceptability than policies designed around progressive taxation and a fairer redistribution of wealth across society. So there are opportunities for the public health community to link its health improvement efforts to this burgeoning interest. For example, Huppert (2005), among others, argues that promoting positive mental health (or psychological well-being) can be a suitable target for population-level interventions. Reducing the mean number of psychological symptoms within a population would enable more individuals to flourish and substantially decrease the number of those meeting the criteria for mental disorder. A range of interventions for improving individual well-being have been tested, through randomized control trials, by the exponents of the positive psychology movement. The principles and practices that have proven successful at the individual level can be made more universally available. A positive mental health agenda therefore represents a win-win situation in which individuals can flourish and society benefit (Huppert 2005).

Over recent years, the public health community has begun to take a much greater interest in the concept of well-being, with this topic providing a focus for an increasing number of national and international public health conferences. Yet this is a complex topic, capable of being defined, understood and measured in very different ways (Carlisle and Hanlon 2007a). So, psychological well-being (which is concerned with good mental functioning, fulfilling one's potential and so on) may be considered an acceptable focus for the public health community, but attention to subjective well-being (positive emotions, happiness and so on) might appear unwarranted, even trivial. The point here is that both types of well-being are important. However, a focus on well-being could still be thought by many in public health to be a confusing and lightweight distraction, an unwanted muddying of the existing waters, or even a serious threat to efforts to achieve greater health equity and social justice (Seedhouse 1995; Cameron et al. 2006). It could, for example, divert policy attention away from topics such as (social) inequalities in health, and towards (individual) well-being.

Good arguments exist to counter such views (Carlisle and Hanlon 2007b). For example, public health has always been a multidisciplinary endeavour encompassing social, political, economic and environmental concerns (Crawshaw 2007) and public health practitioners have long drawn on multidisciplinary forms of knowledge. Nevertheless, the emergence of increasingly specialized forms of knowledge around inequalities risks marginalizing citizen and community knowledge. A genuinely critical public health must take such knowledge seriously: in the broader context of people's lives, well-being may be as legitimate a priority as health, and health itself may not even be a recognized goal at all (Green 2006). Research on well-being in relation to alternative and complementary health practices, for example, highlights the degree to which a focus on well-being enabled people to assert their chosen form of self and identity, regardless of the views of others or their objective conditions (Sointu 2005). So a focus on well-being appropriately places lay knowledge and experience at the heart of a democratic public health movement, and on a par with professional knowledge.

Moreover, many engaged in community health development practice or research now report significant levels of research and intervention 'fatigue' and scepticism around health initiatives and research projects, from the perspective of disadvantaged communities, not least because nothing which really matters to such communities ever seems to change (O'Neill and Williams 2004). An apparently radical public health agenda of tackling structural causes of health inequalities is, in reality, often played out in health promotion policies, community interventions or environmental changes which end up further stigmatizing those whom such policies or interventions were designed to help, or promoting specific health issues at a cost to other, social goals (Green 2006). Efforts to promote well-being may well meet with greater acceptance from disadvantaged groups and communities as it can provide a focus and vehicle for developing collaborative action (Williams et al. 2007). At the international level, Gough et al (2007) suggest that well-being has a valid place in discussions about the complex range of poverties found in the developing world, and they conclude that the concept of well-being is far from irrelevant to work concerned with international development and broader global inequalities.

Well-being and the role of culture

The argument made in the remainder of this chapter is that modern culture – its values, belief systems and assumptions about what constitutes 'the good life' – has a profound impact on well-being that is often underestimated or poorly appreciated by the public health community. But what is 'culture'? Although single definitions remain notoriously elusive, culture can be broadly understood as a system of meanings and symbols that frame the way people in any society perceive the world, locate themselves within this world, and behave in it (Geertz 1973). Cultural influences tend to be perceived in the same way: as the natural order rather than as human constructs that are amenable to change. We create and re-create culture on a daily basis, simply by thinking and acting in ways considered 'normal' in our society. A recent strand of public health research (Eckersley 2006) suggests that mental health and well-being across all modern, Western-type societies are being damaged by particular aspects of contemporary culture:

Economism – this is the tendency to view the world through the lens of economics, to regard a country as an economy rather than a society, and to believe that economic considerations and values are the most important ones.

Materialism and consumerism – this is the attempt to acquire meaning, happiness and fulfilment through the acquisition and the possession of material things. In the modern consumer society, material values rank higher than spiritual values. Non-material aspects of life may be squeezed out.

Individualism – in a highly individualized society, the onus of success in life rests with individuals, as does responsibility for failure. We are subject to the tyranny of excessive choice in life, and of higher expectations which, together with reduced social support and social control, result in a sense of increased risk, uncertainty and insecurity.

Economism, consumerism, materialism and individualism have all become cultural norms of late modernity and have had many important influences on our lives. Together, they sustain our economy and give purpose and meaning to many lives. Multiple consequences for the public's health flow from this, one of which has been a loss of well-being, characterized by our inability to get off the 'hedonic treadmill' of pursuit of short-term pleasure, chronic choice anxiety, poor work–life balance, various forms of addictive behaviour and so on. There is ample evidence that we also live increasingly dissatisfied, anxious and insecure lives (Bauman 1998). As indicated in Chapter 1, there is considerable evidence that people in affluent nations suffer from increasing levels of depression and anxiety (Layard 2006; James 2008) while average levels of well-being, happiness and life satisfaction appear static or in decline (Easterlin 1980; Lane 2000).

Psychologist Daniel Nettle (2005) suggests that expectations of happiness in our society may be unrealistically high, although he acknowledges that this can be hard to accept in a culture obsessed with personal feelings. But for many economists this lack of increase in average happiness is a disturbing paradox in need of explanation. To over-simplify, it throws into doubt some key assumptions about the causal relationship between our objective welfare (the broad conditions in which we live) and our subjective well-being (how happy we are and how good we feel about our lives). It also throws in doubt the validity of 'rational actor theory' – the assumption long held by many economists that human beings are rational actors who maximize their 'utility' (well-being) through making rational choices in life. The more choice we have the better, and choice is in large part facilitated by wealth.

Yet evidence from economic research shows that increases in income, once past a threshold where basic needs are satisfied, produces diminishing returns in *average* levels of well-being (Easterlin 1980). But this is not the same thing as saying that money does not make us happy as individuals. Economic research shows that, within societies, the wealthiest people are happier than the poorest, which supports the fundamental economic position that wealth is a self-evident good because it increases choice and permits the individual to maximize their 'utility' or well-being. The paradox which economist Richard Layard (2006) puts before us is that, when individuals become richer compared with other individuals, they become happier. However, when already affluent societies become even richer, there is very little increase in average levels of well-being. At above roughly $20,000 per head, higher average income within a country is no guarantee of greater happiness for that society. Conversely, in the developing world, increasing income does benefit both objective welfare and subjective well-being.

Evolutionary psychiatrist Nesse (2005) argues that we humans are bio-logically designed to pursue social goals which are not necessarily conducive to our long-term well-being. This is because we adopt the social norms and behavioural strategies of those around us that seem likely to ensure repro-ductive success, rather than well-being. We feel good when successful in pur-suing such strategies. In our society those are likely to include social status, a professional or other good career, the acquisition of luxury goods and so on. This 'positional psychology', which is inherited from our distant evolu-tionary past according to Nesse, leads us to invest in sources of happiness which are intrinsically relative to what others have. Modern society thus creates motivational responses within us that leave many of us possibly sac-rificing much in life in order to pursue social goals which require massive effort, even though their attainment remains uncertain. Worse still, alterna-tives may be few and unsatisfactory, even though the inability to disengage from a major but unreachable life goal is a recipe for serious depression (Nesse 2005).

Economists like Offer (2006) have reached similar conclusions: that we suffer from various kinds of myopia when it comes to our future well-being. Many of the choices we make in the short term are demonstrably short-sighted and fallible when it comes to producing well-being over the longer term. Most people find prudence and self-control extremely difficult and short-term gratification, even addiction, easy: finding a balance may be the key to satisfaction but this is hard to achieve. Offer also finds that the constant flow of new rewards which are readily available to many people in wealthy society actually undermines our capacity to enjoy them. This is the paradox of affluence. If we fail to foresee that we get used to happiness and a sense of well-being derived from, say, material possessions, then we over-invest in acquiring them.

The paradox for public health is that, while much research suggests that Western-type culture is pathological for individual and social well-being, that culture also fulfils particular psychological needs that arise from modern forms of society. Political scientists and sociologists argue that there is enormous cultural pressure on us to consume, in the name of certain contemporary ideals about what constitutes 'the good life' (Hartmut 1998; Ransome 2005). This is not a trivial issue that relates simply to an apparent obsession with shopping and 'retail therapy' in modern society but is central to how we conceive of our selves (Giddens 1991). This is because the widespread social changes that have occurred in the last two hundred years, and particularly during the last century, have resulted in the loss or abandonment of traditional sources of meaning and social values. This means that a sense of self and purpose in life are no longer a 'given' or ascribed at birth, as was the case in earlier forms of society (Featherstone 1991). The development of a sense of self and life's purpose thus becomes a key task for all of us. Consumption practices provide us with meaning, purpose and a way of constructing appropriate personal and social identities (Giddens 1991). This points to the ways in which we seek to solve our contemporary existential crisis, while simultaneously maintaining the modern way of life with all its comforts.

A further implication for public health is that, because wealth is now a marker for status and success, poverty is arguably more stigmatized now than in the past. An inability to acquire the fruits of modern consumer culture may lead to forms of inequality and social exclusion, particularly in the absence of other forms of social belonging. The serious consequences of consumerism in terms of increasing personal debt are well known. Yet it is important not to jump to conclusions about the relationship between economic status and participation in consumer culture, or to assume that there is a straightforward relationship between poverty and exclusion from consumer culture or wealth and inclusion (Lury 2003). While poverty restricts the possibility of participating in consumption *per se*, it does not necessarily prevent participation in consumer culture. On the contrary, it may incite participation despite lack of income, because of the power of possessions and lifestyle practices to convey symbolic rewards: prestige and social honour (Lury 2003).

An integrative framework

Contemporary philosophy provides an unconventional route from the malaise of modern culture and its impact on human well-being, back to public health thinking and practice, in the form of Ken Wilber's Integral Theory (Wilber 2001). This theory provides a useful way of understanding why current public health approaches are not successful in tackling some modern public health challenges, such as the values now embedded in consumer society. This section applies integral theory to the loss of well-being in affluent society, an important public health issue in its own right but one which provides insight into the interconnected problems of modern life (Hanlon et al. 2010). Wilber argues that human experience needs to be considered from two interacting dimensions (Wilber 2001). The first is that of our subjective or interior world and its objective or exterior world counterpart. The second distinguishes between individual and collective levels of experience. Figure 5.1 illustrates this. The two right quadrants are familiar to public health because they utilize scientific and technical knowledge *and* acknowledge the importance of social, political and economic systems. But the two left quadrants still remain fairly unfamiliar territory. Awareness of the upper left quadrant has largely been restricted to models and theories of individual motivation and behaviour change, while little serious attention is paid to the inter-subjective world of the lower left quadrant. So the framework looks rather different, from a conventional public health perspective (see Figure 5.2).

Wilber makes it clear that all four quadrants matter and must be considered together because each influences all the others. Public health cannot afford to leave out or marginalize any of these because forces exerted within

	Subjective-Interior	Objective-Exterior
Individual level	**I** The inner world of the individual: how I think and understand myself; my values; my ethical stance.	**It** The physical body and brain; the results of empirical, objective study of human experience and the physical world that produce scientific evidence.
Collective level	**We** Our inter-subjective or cultural world of learned, shared, beliefs and values; our collective, negotiated and symbolic system of meanings; the basis for our ethics.	**Its** Economies; social structures and hierarchies; organizations; government policies; the world of business, production; eco-systems.

Figure 5.1 Interacting dimensions of human experience.

	Subjective-Interior	Objective-Exterior
Individual level	I	**It** The physical body and brain; the results of empirical, objective study of human experience and the physical world that produce scientific evidence.
Collective level	**We**	**Its** Economies; social structures and hierarchies; organizations; government policies; the world of business, production; ecosystems.

Figure 5.2 Interacting dimensions of human experience – basic public health model.

a neglected dimension can destroy efforts elsewhere. A fictional case study or 'modern parable' can be used to illustrate and explore the influences of those dimensions. The narrative form is useful here because of its capacity to evoke and convey complex, embodied notions and understandings seldom accessible through other means, such as conventional scientific representations of 'truth' (Banks and Banks 1998). The point of using evocative writing is to enable readers to understand the topic from a variety of perspectives, including the personal, and to engage at an emotional level (Abma 2002; Rhodes and Brown 2005).

The brief vignettes described in Box 5.1 hint at some of the pressures we experience in the modern world: poor work–life balance, consumerism, relative poverty, fear of debt, depression, obesity and addiction. These problems of modernity affect poorer people most profoundly but, as our story shows, the rich and seemingly successful are also caught in this web. The parable in Box 5.1 captures the paradoxical ways in which people in affluent societies both suffer from and contribute to the broader human problems which arise from such societies. This 'case' is grounded in theory and evidence from disciplines such as psychology, economics, sociology, anthropology and political science (Bourdieu 1984; Schor 1999; Schwartz 2000; Bauman 2001; Sullivan and Gershuny 2004; Huppert et al. 2005).

Box 5.1 A parable of our times

Travel in your mind's eye to one of our new cathedrals to consumerism: the latest out of town shopping complex. We focus first on Maureen who is there with her 15-year-old son, Chris. He's clad from head to toe in cyclist designer gear and wants a new bike, although he has a fairly new model at home. Chris hangs around with his cycling friends on the steps of the local concert hall where they perform various cycling stunts, attracting admiration from some and irritation from others. So Chris nags his mother for the latest model which carries a price tag of over £500. Maureen tries to persuade her son that he doesn't really need this, but hasn't really got the emotional energy for yet one more confrontation with persistent teenage pester power. Maureen is about to have another major depressive episode, one of many over the years. She's been prescribed Prozac yet again. In many ways Maureen's depression is an appropriate response to her difficult circumstances. She is deeply in debt and recently separated from a husband who is proving to be unreliable in his provision of support. She is desperate not to go further into debt but just can't resist the pressure from her son to buy this expensive bike. Such immediate pressures are not the only causes of Maureen's depression, which also stems from her early life experiences and a whole lifecourse of difficulties and stresses. The burden of debt and recent break-up of the family brings on the current episode but it's the catalyst, not the root cause.

Also in the store today is Alan, a successful lawyer in early middle age. Maureen's teenage son is a conspicuous consumer who likes to parade his purchases – that's largely the point of having them. Alan, however, is what sociologists call 'an inconspicuous consumer'. He, like many other comparatively wealthy people, buys things that represent an ideal in life – even to some extent an ideal of the self – but which nevertheless tend to remain unused. Alan has a good job and a reasonably content marriage but much of his life feels as if it's gone stale. He's constantly busy but gains little satisfaction from his work. He arrives home exhausted each evening and has a drink most nights to help him relax. He eats for comfort, to the point where he knows he's become very overweight. He also worries about his son, with whom he has not spent 'quality time' for several years. Alan dreams about them both going cycling together so he is here to spend £2,000 on a new bike for himself. Yet this bike will sit in his garage, unused, and the dream cycling trip never materializes. His relationship with his son will continue to slowly deteriorate. But the act of purchase in itself convinces Alan, at least for a while, that as he's willing to spend so much on a bike for a holiday with his son, he must be serious about rebuilding the relationship.

At the other end of the store are Sara and her young son, Jamie. Sara is a 'defiant consumer' – someone who is utterly fed up with being told what to do by 'experts'. She smoked and used drugs while pregnant and argued vigorously with her health care providers when they suggested this might not be good for her health or that of her child. Sara is believed to be 'hard to reach' by various professionals involved with her and her son. Her social worker has warned her that Jamie, who is now 6 years old, could be taken away from her for his own protection. For Sara, Jamie is the one thing that really matters to her and she'd be devastated if she lost him. Jamie has his own problems: he's been labelled

(continued)

ADHD, has suffered from a variety of nutritional deficiencies, and spends a great deal of time watching TV and playing video games. Jamie is already obese. Sara can't afford a bike for him but her mother is with them. Jamie's grand-mother is willing to pay for the bike (a considerable financial sacrifice for her) in the hope that he'll go out and play with friends, and maybe lose some weight.

Empty quadrants, missing dimensions

Thinking for the moment of Alan, what results can we plausibly envisage? (The cases of Maureen and Sara are considered in later chapters.) His doctor's recommendations would probably improve his mood but leave deeper issues untouched. Cognitive behavioural therapy (CBT) and other techniques from positive psychology (Seligman et al. 2005) might achieve a similar effect, but this will not necessarily have a lasting impact, or address some of the deeper issues. Psychological therapies can help re-frame our individual perspective on the world but the proliferation of CBT will not, by itself, solve the problems presented here. Alan's lifestyle problems might be influenced by health promotion but as he lacks neither knowledge nor individual power this approach lacks promise. And there are reasons to be cautious in advocating social marketing as a solution. Social marketing campaigns to combat overuse of alcohol, or obesity, may have some impact on individuals, but the advertising and marketing arms of the food and drink industry use far greater sums of money to influence people in other directions.

Policies to help individuals achieve a better work–life balance may contribute to a better social environment, as might work on fostering community empowerment and developing higher levels of social capital. However, because such approaches have provided little conclusive evidence of *comprehensive* change it is not obvious that they would provide a solution. Alan's individual and collective 'interior' remains, in effect, unknown and untouched. The fact is that he enjoys the material, sensory pleasures his salary affords – good food, fine wines and so on. And he's not a 'cultural dope', easily and unthinkingly seduced by the advertising and marketing industry – but he does like indulging his taste for particular consumer goods. In many ways he does appear on the surface to be living 'the good life', certainly a life that many with far less would envy. So any motivation to change things is up against powerful influences to preserve a quasi-desirable *status quo*.

The approaches outlined above suggest that public health needs a better understanding of and capacity to address the subjective and shared influences that shape health and well-being. A fuller understanding of these vital dimensions is a task well beyond the scope of this book, so we limit ourselves to a brief summary here. Many self-improvement approaches have evolved to populate the upper left quadrant of the model shown in Figure 5.1 (the inner self). These include mindfulness practices, yoga, meditation, various forms of martial arts, Tai Chi, psychotherapy, and other routes to self-mastery and self-awareness. But Alan might feel it just too hard to change, for all the reasons outlined above on how culture influences our thinking and practice. It's difficult for him, as an individual, to make the connections between broader social changes in Western nations and associated changes in meanings and values that impact on people's lives. He like many others in modern society, is a calculating consumer (Featherstone 1991): that is, he engages in 'bounded' consumption and is not 'out of control' in any area of his life (Brain 2002). The pleasures of consumption and the search for instant gratification are, arguably, the rewards for the self-control, restraint and self-management required to steer our individual biographies through the complex world of modern society.

For public health, the point of Wilber's model is that it highlights enduring disciplinary blind-spots: public health may acknowledge the existence of 'culture' as a potential determinant of health and well-being (Carlisle et al. 2008) but is normally silent about either the role of sensory pleasure in creating some types of health problems, or the transformative potential of 'inner work' in tackling them. Whilst the complex problems outlined above will not be solved simply by paying more attention to lesser-known dimensions, the influence of forces from those dimensions can certainly undermine or even destroy public health efforts in familiar fields. The strength of integral theory – conceived in terms of an integrative approach to public health – is its emphasis that all key dimensions of human experience need to be considered, harmonized and acted on *as a whole*. Public health as a discipline has not yet fully reached this level of understanding; and there is also the larger question of how best we can act, when we do reach it.

Conclusions

Understanding the sources and causes of cultural problems requires the public health community to look well beyond the already broad boundaries of public health, in order to draw on the insights of other relevant disciplines, such as psychology, economics, sociology and anthropology. Insights from these disciplines reveal that few of us are fully aware of the ways in which the cultural belief systems, values and assumptions associated with the modern capitalist economy can influence our choices, or of how much those choices contribute to the sense we have of ourselves and our purpose in life, and the broader implications for our health and well-being. Expressed in this way, a concern with well-being and happiness is not a trivial issue, and thus

irrelevant to public health. Longer-term well-being is known to be strongly associated with good personal and social relationships, fulfilling and rewarding
forms of work, worthwhile forms of leisure activities, together with a sense of
freedom *and* security.

Yet even within the neo-liberal economies of Western societies the search
for well-being can resist commodified or consumerist forms, as demonstrated
by various New Social Movements motivated by ecological concerns or equity
advocacy, or the rise in 'downshifters', for example (Hamilton 2003). Increasing numbers of people seem aware of the downside of over-consumption,
which involves more than rising levels of personal debt and bankruptcy and
is implicated in the kinds of planetary climate change likely to hit the poorest
nations of the world hardest, as described in Chapter 8. A focus on well-being
therefore has the potential to subvert the interests of the market by rejecting
some of the more damaging cultural norms associated with the neo-liberal
economies. For public health, a fuller understanding of well-being as a key
component of our individual and social quality of life, and the ways in which
it can be influenced, manipulated and distorted by market forces, can help
in the pursuit of greater social and global equity – an argument made in
Chapter 4 and pursued in greater depth in Chapter 8.

There is also the argument that unfettered, individualized freedom
of choice can undermine social attempts to consider appropriate levels of
consumption. In the context of emergent concerns with environmental
sustainability, the question of appropriate *social* levels of consumption
seems an increasingly urgent task. Economic activities in any society, when
unchecked, can overwhelm the physical life support systems on this planet
so some philosophers have argued that it is rational to limit individual and
social consumption in order to protect the systems on which global humanity
depends (Cafaro 2001). Although public health is not necessarily comfortable
with the question 'how should we live?', the arguments rehearsed in this
chapter suggest that what we take to be the good life, and what we believe
contributes to human well-being, need to be re-thought. This is a task for
public health as much as for any other discipline: our existing scientific base,
our ability to grasp and use relevant knowledge from other fields, and our
capacity for advocacy in the cause of health and well-being all indicate that
we may be uniquely placed to pursue it.

References

Abma, T.A. (2002) Emerging narrative forms of knowledge representation in the
    health sciences: two texts in a postmodern context. *Qualitative Health Research*,
    2: 5–27.
Banks, A. and Banks, S. (1998) *Fiction and Social Research: By Ice or Fire*. Walnut
    Creek, CA: AltaMira Press.

Bauman, Z. (1998) *Work, Consumerism and the New Poor*. Buckingham: Open University Press.

Bauman, Z. (2000) *Liquid Modernity*. Cambridge: Polity Press.

Bauman, Z. (2001) *The Individualized Society*. Cambridge: Polity Press.

Bourdieu, P. (1984) *Distinction: A Social Critique of the Judgement of Taste*. London: Routledge.

Brain, K. (2002) Youth, Alcohol and the Emergence of the Post Modern Alcohol Order. London: Occasional Paper, Institute of Alcohol Studies. http://www.ias.org.uk/resources/nighttime/literature/enactments.html (accessed 17 September 2011)

Cafaro, P. (2001) Economic consumption, pleasure, and the good life. *Journal of Social Philosophy*, 32: 471–86.

Cameron, E., Mathers, J. and Parry, J. (2006) 'Health and well-being': questioning the use of health concepts in public health policy and practice. *Critical Public Health*, 16: 347–54.

Carlisle, S. and Hanlon P. (2007a) The complex territory of well-being: contestable evidence, contentious theories and speculative conclusions. *Journal of Public Mental Health*, 6: 8–13.

Carlisle, S. and Hanlon, P. (2007b) Well-being and consumer culture: a different kind of public health problem? *Health Promotion International*, 22(3): 261–8.

Carlisle, S., Hanlon, P. and Hannah, M. (2008) Status, taste and distinction in consumer culture: acknowledging the symbolic dimensions of inequality. *Public Health*, 122: 631–7.

Carlisle, S., Henderson, G. and Hanlon, P. (2009) 'Wellbeing': a collateral casualty of modernity? *Social Science and Medicine*, 69: 1556–60.

Crawshaw, P. (2007) For a multidisciplinary public health (editorial). *Critical Public Health*, 17: 1–2.

CSDH (Commission on the Social Determinants of Health) (2008) *Closing the Gap in a Generation: Health Equity Through Action on the Social Determinants of Health*. Final Report of the Commission on Social Determinants of Health. Geneva: World Health Organization.

Easterlin, R.A. (1980) Does economic growth improve the human lot? Some empirical evidence. *Social Indicators Research*, 8: 199–221.

Eckersley, R. (2006) Is modern Western culture a health hazard? *International Journal of Epidemiology*, 35: 252–8.

Featherstone, M. (1991) *Consumer Culture and Postmodernism*. London: Sage.

Fukuyama, F. (1999) *The Great Disruption: Human Nature and the Reconstitution of Social Order*. New York: Free Press.

Geertz, C. (1973) *The Interpretation of Cultures*. New York: Basic Books.

Giddens, A. (1991) *Modernity and Self-identity: Self and Society in the Late Modern Age*. Cambridge: Polity Press.

Gough, I., McGregor, J.A. and Camfield, L. (2007) Theorising wellbeing in international development. In I. Gough and J.A. McGregor (eds) *Wellbeing in Developing Countries: From Theory to Research*. Cambridge: Cambridge University Press.

Gould, N. and Gould, E. (2001) Health as a consumption object: research notes and preliminary investigation. *International Journal of Consumer Studies*, 25(2): 90–101.

Green, J. (2006) What role for critical public health? *Critical Public Health*, 16: 171–3.

Hamilton, C. (2003) *Downshifting in Britain: A Sea-change in the Pursuit of Happiness*. Discussion Paper 58. Melbourne: The Australia Institute.

Hanlon, P. and Carlisle, S. (2010) Re-orienting public health: rhetoric, challenges and possibilities for sustainability. *Critical Public Health*, 20(3): 299–309.

Hanlon, P., Carlisle, S., Reilly, D., Lyon, A. and Hannah, M. (2010) Enabling well-being in a time of radical change: integrative public health for the 21st century. *Public Health*, 124: 305–12.

Hartmut, R. (1998) On defining the good life: liberal freedom and capitalist necessity. *Constellations*, 5(2): 201–14.

Himmelfarb, G. (2008) *The Roads to Modernity: The British, French and American Enlightenments*. London: Vintage.

Huppert, F.A. (2005) Positive mental health in individuals and populations. In F.A. Huppert, N. Bayliss and B. Keverne (eds) *The Science of Well-Being*. Oxford: Oxford University Press.

Huppert, F.A., Baylis, N. and Keverne, B. (eds) (2005) *The Science of Well-Being*. Oxford: Oxford University Press.

Intergovernmental Panel on Climate Change (1996) *Second Assessment Report*. New York: Cambridge University Press.

Intergovernmental Panel on Climate Change (2007) *Fourth Assessment Report*. New York: Cambridge University Press.

James, O. (2008) *The Selfish Capitalist*. London: Vermilion.

Lane, R.E. (2000) *The Loss of Happiness in Market Democracies*. London: Yale University Press.

Layard, R. (2006) *Happiness: Lessons from a New Science*. Harmondsworth: Penguin Books.

Lury, C. (2003) *Consumer Culture*. Cambridge: Polity Press.

Marmot Review (2010) *Fair Society, Healthy Lives. Strategic Review of Inequalities in Health in England Post-2010* (Chair: Sir Michael Marmot). London: University College London.

Nesse, R.M. (2005) Natural selection and the elusiveness of happiness. In F.A. Huppert, N. Baylis and B. Keverne (eds) *The Science of Well-being*. Oxford: Oxford University Press.

Nettle, D. (2005) *The Science Behind Your Smile*. Oxford: Oxford University Press.

Offer, A. (2006) *The Challenge of Affluence: Self Control and Well-being in the United States and Britain Since 1950*. Oxford: Oxford University Press.

O'Neil, M. and Williams, G. (2004) Developing community and agency engagement in an action research study in South Wales. *Critical Public Health*, 14: 37–48.

Pahl, R. (1998) The Social Context of Healthy Living. London: The Nuffield Trust.

Ransome, P. (2005) *Work, Consumption and Culture: Affluence and Social Change in the 21st Century*. London: Sage.

Rhodes, C. and Brown, A.D. (2005) Writing responsibly: narrative fiction and organization studies. *Organization*, 12: 467–91

Roberts, B. (2005) *The End of Oil*. London: Bloomsbury.

Schor, J. (1999) *The Overspent American: Why we want what we don't need*. New York: Harper Perennial.

Schwartz, B. (2000) Self-determination: the tyranny of freedom. *American Psychologist*, 55: 79–88.

Seedhouse, D. (1995) Well-being: health promotion's red herring. *Health Promotion International*, 10: 61–7.

Seligman, M.E.P., Parks, A.C. and Steen, T. (2005) A balanced psychology and a full life. In F.A. Huppert, N. Baylis and B. Keverne (eds) *The Science of Well-being*. Oxford: Oxford University Press.

Sointu, E. (2005) The rise of an ideal: tracing changing discourses of well-being. *Sociological Review*, 53: 255–74.

Sullivan, O. and Gershuny, J. (2004) Inconspicuous consumption: work-rich, time-poor in the liberal market economy. *Journal of Consumer Culture*, 4: 79–100.

Wilber, K. (2001) *A Theory of Everything: An Integral Vision for Business, Politics, Science and Spirituality*. Dublin: Gateway.

Wilkinson, R. and Pickett, K. (2009) *The Spirit Level: Why More Equal Societies Almost Always do Better*. London: Allen Lane.

Williams, G., Cropper, S., Porter, A. et al. (2007) *Community Health and Wellbeing: Action Research on Health Inequalities*. Bristol: Policy Press.

Wilmott, M. and Nelson, W. (2005) *Complicated Lives: The Malaise of Modernity*. Chichester: John Wiley & Sons.

World Health Organization (2001) *Mental Health: New Understanding, New Hope*. Geneva: World Health Organization.

World Health Organization (2005) *Promoting Mental Health: Concepts, Emerging Evidence, Practice*. Geneva: World Health Organization.

6 Modern public health challenges – obesity and addiction

Introduction

This chapter examines two public health challenges of modern society which are, apparently, deepening: obesity and various forms of addiction (to drugs and alcohol in particular). Their observed increase is often referred to as an 'epidemic', not because either is caused by infectious agents but because they appear to be steadily rising in frequency from historically low baseline levels. They also appear to be particularly resistant to tried-and-tested public health approaches, such as the provision of healthy lifestyle information, community-level interventions, or primary care-led initiatives. To focus on obesity and addiction is not in any way equivalent to suggesting that long-standing public health problems such as ischaemic heart disease, stroke or cancer have suddenly become irrelevant to the public health community. Improvements in prevention and treatment in those areas have been made over recent decades, but public health practitioners rightly continue to focus their efforts on these and other significant health conditions.

In the context of the arguments made in this book, however, obesity and various forms of addictive behaviour bear particularly close examination. This is partly because of their relationship to late industrial society and its culture (the nature of which was explored to some extent in Chapter 5). But it is also because they exemplify the ways in which emerging public health problems are no longer capable of resolution via the 'understand, predict and control' approach (and mindset) which has formerly been so useful in public health practice. Many working in public health may feel there is an intuitive – even an obvious – link between the behaviours that contribute to obesity and various addictions (to alcohol, tobacco or recreational drugs, for example). The argument made in this chapter is not that individual behaviour has no contribution to make to weight gain or addiction-related health problems: it is rather that the type of society we live in and the cultural assumptions we live by are at least as influential as any individual choice. Such issues are explored below.

Obesity

Obesity is rising across the world (Nishida et al. 2002). In 2006, the number of obese and overweight people in the world overtook the numbers who are malnourished and underweight (Popkin 2009). Obesity is quite simply a condition characterized by an excess of body fat. There are a variety of ways in which obesity can be assessed in individuals and populations (Seidell and Flegal 1997). One commonly used definition of obesity is the body mass index (BMI), which is a person's weight in kilograms divided by the square of their height in metres. For adults, overweight is defined as a BMI of greater than 25 and obesity is defined as a BMI of greater than 30. This definition is not entirely unproblematic, as an athlete with a large muscle bulk can have a high BMI but not be obese. Waist circumference, waist/hip ratio and skin fold thickness are alternative assessment tools. The standard BMI classification is:

BMI range (kg/m^2)	Classification
< 17	Malnourished
17–<20	Underweight
20–<25	Normal weight
25–<30	Overweight
30–<40	Obese

The terms overweight and obese are mutually exclusive when using BMI, so the category of overweight does not include obese. Most wealthy nations are experiencing an epidemic of obesity (Sassi et al. 2009). The medical response has been to focus attention on those who are obese, to debate whether being overweight is really a problem, and to ignore those in the normal BMI category. However, the rise in obesity has resulted from a marked shift in the whole population towards a greater BMI, rather than from a smaller number of individuals becoming heavier. So the slim are becoming less slim while the already overweight are getting heavier, and the number of people in the obese category steadily grows. This shift in weight distribution translates into a one kilogram increase in weight per adult per year (on average over the adult population). The increase cannot be accounted for simply by an ageing population. The consequence of this trend is that the UK has one of the highest levels of obesity in OECD countries, following the United States of America (Sassi et al. 2009).

The health risks of obesity are serious (Wright et al. 2001). People who are obese are more likely to develop a range of chronic conditions, including osteoarthritis, high blood pressure, diabetes, heart disease and some cancers.

Children are not immune from these risks. They are particularly vulnerable to social and environmental pressures that increase the risk of obesity. Until recently, type 2 diabetes was only seen in adults, but now some adolescents are developing this condition. This can lead in later life to serious consequences such as heart disease, stroke, kidney failure and blindness. Nor are the effects limited to physical illnesses. For example, obese children (especially girls) are more likely to show evidence of psychological distress than children who are not obese (Braet et al. 1997). The prevalence of obesity (BMI greater than 30) in the UK has increased since the early 1980s. In 2008, almost a quarter of adults (24 per cent of men and 25 per cent of women aged 16 or over) in England were classified as obese (BMI 30 kg/m^2 or over). A greater proportion of men than women (42 per cent compared with 32 per cent) in England were classified as overweight in 2008 (BMI 25 to less than 30 kg/m^2) (NHS Information Centre: Lifestyle Statistics 2010). Obesity is now common in children: nearly 1 in 5 (18 per cent) of boys and 1 in 10 (14 per cent) of girls aged 2 to 15 years are obese.

Obesogenic organisms in an obesogenic environment

As noted in the introduction to this chapter, it is now widely accepted that the current obesity epidemic cannot be blamed on individual behaviour and poor choice, notwithstanding the ways this is often represented by the media. Many current approaches, however, still focus on individuals, emphasizing education about diet and exercise and encouraging weight loss. This is in part understandable as, from a purely biological point of view, whether or not each of us becomes obese depends on the balance between our energy input and output. Our bodies have sophisticated mechanisms that can regulate body weight by adjusting energy intake to match energy expenditure and vice versa. However, a more helpful way to understand the current obesity epidemic is to consider humans as obesogenic organisms who, for the first time in their history, find themselves in an obesogenic environment: that is, one where people's routine and everyday circumstances encourage them to eat more and exercise less.

This environment includes the availability of cheap and heavily marketed energy-rich foods, the increase in labour saving devices (such as lifts and re-mote controls) and the massive increase in passive forms of transport (cars as opposed to walking, cycling or walking to public transport hubs). Economic growth in developed and, increasingly, in developing countries has led to a number of social trends which have helped to create this obesogenic en-vironment. The problem is that human physiology was formed long ago in our evolutionary history when food was scarce and we needed large amounts of energy in order to find food and stay alive. Our ancestors are estimated to have expended about 1000 calories per day in physical activity. Human beings adapted to these circumstances by eating food whenever it was available and conserving energy by moving only when necessary. This capacity to store and conserve energy was – and remains – a successful survival strategy in times of scarcity. It is far less helpful in affluent countries, where most of us now live in societies where food is easily come by, and the average sedentary person only expends about 300 calories day in physical activity. We are apparently burdened with the metabolic and behavioural legacy of our evolutionary history – programmed to eat when we can and preserve energy whenever possible. It is therefore not surprising that obesogenic organisms should have problems coping with an environment that exerts constant (but often subtle) pressure to increase energy intake and to decrease energy expenditure. The rise in obesity suggests that, for more and more people, the effects of our obesogenic environment are overriding our biological regulatory mechanisms.

Public health approaches

It has become an axiom of health promotion that we should try to create supportive environments in which healthier choices are made the easier choices (World Health Organization 1986). We have therefore tried to move from solutions focused on individual people towards making changes to our physical and social environments, while encouraging people to eat more wisely and expend more energy. We have tried offering free fruit in schools, improving labelling on foods, providing free swimming for children, and building cycle paths, to name only a few environmentally-focused initiatives. It is theoretically possible that changes to the environment could shift the behaviour of large numbers of people and prevent them from gaining weight if the changes were large enough. But it is also the case that many of the adjustments we have tried to make to our environment have, in reality, been quite marginal, as the obesity statistics make clear. Obesity is a worrying example of our failure to understand the nature of the problem, predict and control its course, and provide an appropriate solution.

The multiple levels at which we need to understand the cause of obesity in populations is illustrated by the following simplified list:

- At the cellular level obesity results from the deposition of fat which is under complex biochemical and hormonal control.
- The amount of fat deposition is determined by the balance between energy intake and expenditure at the level of the individual.
- Energy balance is determined by the calories taken in (as food and drink) and calories expended.
- A variety of genetic, psycho-social and other factors operate at the level of the individual to influence consumption and activity.

- Individuals function within settings like the home, school, community and workplace. These settings influence food intake and physical activity.
- There are several levels of organization above these settings that are important. These include the food and drink industry, agriculture, education, the media, the government and its policies, public health, health care, transport and recreation.
- Cultural influences have an effect that pervades many settings, structures and policies.

Two points flow from this analysis. First, effective strategies to combat obesity may be needed at all these levels. Second, the factors that influence obesity are also important for other aspects of health that are creating patterns of obesity in whole populations. Modelling work carried out by the USA Centers for Disease Control and Prevention suggests that only strategies that impact on all age groups will reverse the obesity epidemic (Centers for Disease Control and Prevention 2010). This, combined with an understanding of the determinants of obesity, suggests that population-based strategies will have to confront all age groups and influence all levels. What might be required for the UK includes:

- International action directed at the production of food;
- European Union policies which will impact upon agriculture and transport;
- UK legislation (for example to control food advertising to children);
- Interventions designed to influence the key settings described above;
- Specific actions to combat the obesogenic environment (vending machines in schools, recreation activities, outlets for food and so on);
- Initiatives directed towards individuals to help them to avoid gaining weight;
- Initiatives directed towards those who are overweight and obese to help them lose weight;
- Actions by components of civic society to influence cultural norms and mores, beliefs and assumptions.

Such an approach might be called an 'all ages, all levels' strategy, and reflects the thinking of both the 'Health for All' and evidence-based public health movements described in Chapter 3. Yet the lack of success from current approaches, as indicated by the worsening statistics on obesity, suggests that the challenge remains profound and will require new ways of thinking and practice.

Applying integrative understanding to obesity

Chapter 5 provided a set of vignettes (see Box 5.1) of the types of problems that beset many people in 'modern' society. In this modern tale, Jamie was a young boy with a number of health problems, including obesity. The difficult life circumstances of his family suggest that losing weight may not be a high priority for him or for Sara, his mother. Alan, the successful lawyer, has a poor level of well-being that is in part manifested through overeating. Sara, Jamie's mother, and Maureen (mother of teenage cycle enthusiast Chris) are also overweight and will, in several years (if current weight gain trends continue), become obese. What help can any of them be offered from the current health care system or from health promotion expertise? The integrative approach described in Chapter 5 can be applied here.

The initial response of the health care system will probably be similar for all four, child and adults. The main message will be 'eat more healthily and take more exercise' – a message transmitted to Jamie through school-based programmes, and to the adults through social marketing campaigns. Specific support from a dietician may be offered to Sara, as she has contact with several health and social care professionals, to help with her and Jamie's diet. However, Sara is not likely to pay much attention to the dietician, who appears to be just one more interfering professional telling her how to live her life and raise her child. Alan already knows all the health 'messages', has been on a multitude of diets, and even employed a personal trainer for several months. These strategies worked for a while but he always put back on all the weight he lost, and often more. And Maureen, who is bordering on a depressive episode, is not likely to have the emotional energy or motivation to embark on yet one more weight-loss programme: she's been there, done that, and 'bought the T-shirt' many times before.

Policy makers are well aware of the influence of the obesogenic environment, described in reports like that compiled by the Foresight group (Foresight Report 2007). Many politicians across the political spectrum still appear to believe that personal responsibility for living healthily is still under-emphasized. However, the influence and power of food manufacturers and large supermarket chains is such that only marginal changes are made. Many local public health and/or health promotion initiatives have also tried to address the problem of the obesogenic environment. Figure 6.1 uses the integral framework to summarize just some of the existing responses to the obesity epidemic (shown in the right hand quadrants of the diagram). It also highlights the forces ranged against them, in terms of individual and collective influences (the left hand quadrants of the diagram).

	Interior-Subjective	**Exterior-Objective**
Individual level	**I** Many individuals respond to social and medical pressure to lose weight by engaging in weight-loss programmes of many forms, sometimes over many years. Yet the 'problem' never seems to disappear for good and 'yo-yo' dieting has become a feature of many individual lives. Food is rarely (if ever) understood at the individual level purely as 'fuel'. Food is a source of sensory pleasure and enjoyment for nearly everyone. Food also has multiple, *social* meanings that all individuals draw on in their eating choices. For example, food can be used to demonstrate love and care for others, or gratitude. It can be used for sensual pleasure and gratification, for celebration with others, for ritual purposes, or for comfort and solace (of self and others) during low points in life. Food can convey social status and 'good taste'. It can be deployed as part of the 'art of seduction'. And so on ...	**It** A substantial body of high quality nutritional research exists, so much is known about what constitutes a healthy daily diet for men, women and children across the various stages of the lifecourse. With regard to a healthy weight, calories in and calories out (increasing physical activity) is the main focus. From this objective perspective, food is understood primarily as fuel for physiological maintenance and effective functioning.
Collective level	**We** Collectively, we are targets for extremely well-funded and sophisticated food and drink advertising and marketing campaigns. The multiple social and cultural meanings associated with food (briefly listed above), and its many pleasures, are successfully manipulated by organizations, industries and individuals who stand to make a profit. Fat and sugar content *changes* in food are successfully resisted by the food and drink industry. Conversely, we are also aware that being overweight is neither socially nor medically desirable, so there is a considerable market in persuading us that we need various slimming and/or exercise products, to counter the marketing successes achieved elsewhere!	**Its** Advice on healthy eating and exercise is freely available from many sources. Adults are encouraged to take responsibility for their choices and to make necessary changes. Exercise on prescription may be offered, such as free gym or swimming passes. Local initiatives aimed at children may include a 'walk to school' campaign and attempts to reduce fast food outlets near schools. Families may be encouraged to grow some fruit and vegetables, and allotments are increasingly available. Policy makers ensure that salt in some manufactured foods is reduced and nutritional content (including amount of fat and sugar) is labelled.

Figure 6.1 Understanding the four dimensions of obesity.

Implications for public health

It is clear that our biology does matter, in terms of appetite control, exercise, drives and so on, and the knowledge and interventions referred to in the right hand column of Figure 6.1 (the objective, exterior quadrants of the model) are significant. Yet it seems implausible that they will outweigh the influences suggested by the left hand column, which deals with our subjective, interior, individual and collective understanding, and the things that influence these. It is not that the individual/subjective quadrant is unimportant: politicians and others are not mistaken when they say that individuals do have the capacity (agency) for making positive change. Nevertheless, although some individuals appear able to resist the forces of an obesogenic environment, the majority of us apparently do not. The point for public health is that the inner world of the individual is complex and is in relationship to the other three quadrants.

The structure of our society (the way it promotes passive forms of transport, for example, and makes cheap sources of calories so ubiquitously available) is also important. Social marketing for health is overwhelmed by superior budgets and highly sophisticated marketing expertise in the food retail sector. The bottom left quadrant is equally important. The culture of consumption discussed in Chapter 5 clearly has a profound influence on our eating behaviour: the nature of our consumer society promotes the obesity epidemic. This suggests that while all four quadrants continue to manifest factors that promote obesity, and interact with each other, there is little prospect of the obesity epidemic being reversed. Many of us will continue to struggle with the problem.

If food is seen primarily as a commodity, the use of which is only to be determined by the market, then regulation and taxation will not be enough. If it is seen purely in nutritional terms, as 'fuel' for the body, then we will remain seriously under-informed about its individual, social and cultural significance (Counihan 1999; Mintz and Du Bois 2002), the true complexity of which cannot be addressed here. If we are treated as consumers where choice is the paramount consideration, rather than citizens with a shared stake in the future, progress will be slow and marginal. While we operate an economy that externalizes the true cost of food miles and wasted food, economic forces will continue to operate in the wrong direction. And as long as social marketing is employed as the main public health tool for engagement with each person's individual and cultural life, then the debate about these problems will remain at the superficial level.

There are those in public health who argue that we need to do for obesity what we have done for smoking. In Chapter 3 we briefly described how smoking prevalence in the UK declined over several decades under the influence of a wide variety of public health interventions which seem to have worked synergistically. So, we might argue, the obesity epidemic could be reversed by taxing fat, regulating the food industry, promoting active commuting, re-designing our cities, employing smart social marketing and making better use of health care interventions. Such strategies may well have some degree of success, but they are unlikely to be sufficient as the obesity epidemic (like the loss of well-being) is an *emergent property* of the modern society in which we live.

There is another point to the tobacco control story that is relevant to obesity but often overlooked. In many affluent societies smoking has now become an 'anti-social' form of behaviour, practised by a minority and stig-matized by many. This has been a cultural shift, and cannot be traced solely to public health influences, actions and interventions. So there is some dan-ger that efforts to tackle obesity can result in the unintended consequence of stigmatizing whole sections of society. We may all need to develop a health-ier relationship to food, which means discovering other ways of dealing with the stresses of life that lead us to use certain kinds of food as solace and comfort, and finding other types of reward systems. We could, for example, turn to forms of practice (such as yoga, mindfulness meditation, and so on) to develop greater self-awareness and capacity for resisting external collective in-fluences. Such interior/subjective changes would be helpful but are unlikely, by themselves, to suffice in tackling the problem.

Addiction

In the field of addictions, terminology is complex and disputed and many models of addiction exist (West 1997). For the purposes of this chapter we employ that developed by psychologist Bruce Alexander (Alexander 2008). He argues that addiction can best be understood as an overwhelming involve-ment with a particular behaviour, such as alcohol or drug consumption. The definition can also, of course, encompass other forms of behaviour which become an overwhelming part of an individual's life, such as gambling, shop-ping, sex, work and so on. The key points for public health are that such over-whelming involvement is an adaptation to psychological distress created by social, cultural and economic circumstances, and that adverse consequences follow, for the overwhelmed individual or for others (Alexander 2008).

Addiction and social disruption

Each individual with a drug or alcohol problem has their own story of how they arrived at that point. Alexander's work, however, looks to a broader social history to discover what circumstances give rise to high rates of over-whelming involvement. He has found that rising problems with addiction are associated with decline and disruption in society as a whole: the converse is also true – addictions are less of a problem during periods when societies are more stable and cohesive (Alexander 2008). Two examples illustrate this general point: addictions are known to have become more of a problem as the Roman Empire moved into decline, and when the indigenous tribal peoples of North America were placed in reservations. Others have made similar observations. For example, alcohol related problems worsened when the Soviet Empire collapsed (Bobak and Marmot 1994). They also worsened when the industrial revolution disrupted the lives of many in Europe during the nineteenth century.

Durkheim (one of the founders of modern sociology) explored what happened to people who were forced out of small agricultural villages and into the cities of the industrial revolution (Durkheim 1897/1952). His research led him to develop the concept of 'anomie', a term used to describe the breakdown of social and moral norms that often follows periods of economic and social change (Durkheim 1897/1952). Anomie is sometimes translated as 'loss of meaning'. Durkheim argued that such change can bring about less regulated societies, in which previous social norms no longer apply and no longer control the behaviour of individuals. The resulting anomie, the loss of perceived purpose and meaning in life, leads to increasing levels of crime and 'deviant' forms of behaviour, including addictions. Durkheim viewed suicide as an extreme manifestation of a more generalized set of self-destructive behaviours. The concept of anomie has also been used to explain why the socio-economic disruption precipitated by the collapse of the USSR led directly to deteriorating health in ex-Communist countries (most notably Russia) from the early 1990s onwards (McKee and Leon 2005). This analysis has highlighted the reduction in life expectancy, the widening of inequalities in life expectancy between regions, and the striking impact of substance misuse, especially alcohol related harm, among men. McKee and Leon found that those who experienced the most rapid and uncontrolled transition, and had least social support, suffered most (McKee and Leon 2005). So Durkheim's work, and that of others who have used his insights, remains an important reminder for public health: individual behaviour should not be examined, and cannot properly be understood, in isolation from social influences.

What similar social influences are at work in the UK today? In the past half century, many parts of the country (South Wales, the North East and the North West of England, parts of the Midlands, Northern Ireland and West Central Scotland) have undergone a transition to become post-industrial regions. This can be illustrated by a few examples. In 1970, nearly 40 per cent of Northern Ireland's workforce was employed in shipbuilding, textiles and other manufactured goods, but by 2005 this had fallen to less than 24 per cent. The miners' strike in 1984 had a devastating effect on the coal industry of South Wales with employment in that industry falling from 220,000 to

7,000 in two decades. Between 1971 and 2005, the West of Scotland shed almost two-thirds (62 per cent) of its jobs in industry, making it one of the most rapidly and profoundly deindustrialized areas of Europe. These trends altered many aspects of life including the family, work, leisure, beliefs, values and norms. In this context it is informative to examine trends in alcohol related harm and drug misuse in recent years. Few can doubt that there is a particular problem in the UK. When compared with the UK, countries like the Netherlands, Sweden, Norway, Australia and New Zealand all have broadly similar cultures, genetic backgrounds and drinking cultures, and in 1986 they had broadly similar liver disease death rates (Sheron et al. 2011). The most recent liver disease death rates for these countries range from 2.6 per 100,000 (New Zealand) to 5.3 (Sweden). In the UK, however, death rates from liver disease more than doubled from 4.9 per 100,000, to 11.4 since 1986 (WHO 2011). And of all the countries in the UK, Scotland has a particular problem with drugs. Statistics reported by the United Nations show that Scotland is the sixth worst country for illicit drug use in the world (United Nations Office on Drugs and Crime 2010). No other comparable country is anywhere near as high in the rankings: Scotland finds itself sixth in the list, behind Afghanistan, Iran, Mauritius, Costa Rica and Russia.

'Addictive societies'?

Alexander argues that although the free-market societies of North America, Australasia and the UK have been extremely productive, they also subject people to irresistible pressures towards individualism and competition, tearing rich and poor alike from the close social and even spiritual ties that normally constitute important parts of human life (Alexander 2008). People adapt to such dislocation by finding the best substitute that they can: addiction serves this function all too well. From public health research, Wilkinson's substantial body of work on inequality over several decades contributes to this set of findings (Wilkinson 1996; Wilkinson and Pickett 2009). This demonstrates that unequal societies are bad for almost everyone within them, the well-off and the poor. Almost every modern health and social problem, including drug and alcohol use, is more likely to occur in a less equal society. The UK is one of the most unequal of the societies analysed by Wilkinson, and also suffers one of the highest rates of drug use.

In summary, researchers in public health and other disciplines have demonstrated that, in societies that have seen considerable growth in trends commonly associated with free markets (such as consumerism, individualism, competition and inequality), people may experience various kinds of individual/psychological and social dislocation. Addictive behaviour is a common adaptive response to such dislocations. The point for public health is that, in societies like the UK, we need to understand addiction as an individual's adaptation – a logical response by the person – to their circumstances, and not an illogical maladaptation. The addicted person, from this perspective, finds in their addiction an appropriate response to the psychological and social dislocation produced by late modern society.

Applying integrative understanding to addiction

Much is known about the existence of drug and alcohol addiction in the UK, as well as about less problematic levels of use. Yet all attempts to reduce problems arising from drugs and alcohol appear subject to the ingenuity gap described in the introduction to this book: that there is a gulf between current problems and the availability of solutions. The problems of drugs and alcohol are confronted in the UK by four linked policy initiatives: prevention, harm reduction, treatment and law enforcement. Each component has value and there are frequent calls for more resources to support them. For alcohol, action on cost and availability has proven to be of value (Jernigan et al. 2000). This has led to calls for such measures to be introduced in the UK (Sheron et al. 2011). Nevertheless, action on price and availability that fails to confront cultural influences as well may not be enough. And despite all these efforts the problem is growing and the ingenuity gap (Homer-Dixon 2000) is all too observable.

A plausible conclusion is that the continuing growth in overwhelming involvement in drugs and alcohol is due to an escalation of social conditions that lead people to adapt to psychological and social dislocation through addictive behaviour. Moreover, drugs and alcohol use are only two manifestations of a more general set of addictive behaviours. If we include the use of overwhelming involvement in gambling, shopping, work and sex then it becomes clear that the problem is very large indeed. In the short story given in Chapter 5 (Box 5.1) Sara was briefly portrayed as someone whose addictive behaviour is, at least in part, a response to her difficult life history and circumstances. How well do current approaches to addiction match her needs, or reflect the analysis set out above? Figure 6.2 uses the four quadrant integrative model introduced in Chapter 4 to identify probable responses (see the right hand quadrants), made in light of current knowledge and understanding of 'what works' (or, perhaps, what is available and affordable). The left hand quadrants illustrates a few tiny examples of how addiction might be experienced by the individual, and perceived in the wider culture – dimensions to which public health has given comparatively little attention.

A key point to make is that, compared to alcohol, there is sometimes even less provision for drugs. For example, methadone 'works', in that it can stabilize the life of a drug user, sometimes for long periods. However, we tend to rely on methadone maintenance to the detriment of other approaches, such as residential rehabilitation, employment, education and recovery. It is only

	Interior-Subjective	Exterior-Objective
Individual level	**I** Alcohol and/or drug consumption is a pleasurable experience for many individuals. For some, excessive consumption represents a rational and meaningful response to difficult, sometimes intolerable, life circumstances, leading to the problem of overwhelming involvement with the substance and neglect of other aspects of life.	**It** Much research has demonstrated the potential for damage to mental and physical health from problematic levels of alcohol or drug use. Methadone maintenance is offered, together with support from drugs workers.
Collective level	**We** Limited use of some drugs and most forms of alcohol is a matter of individual choice and a non-problematic part of life for considerable numbers of people. Problematic levels of drug and alcohol use are largely perceived, by the unaffected majority, as 'other people's problems'. Harsher judgements are also possible, encouraged by some elements of the public media and policy community.	**Its** Programmes for detoxification, rehabilitation and employment are funded. Some drugs are prohibited and their possession and use is illegal. Minimum 'unit' pricing may be recommended for alcohol. Some drugs and most forms of alcohol remain freely available and affordable across society. Their production, marketing and distribution are a source of considerable income for the industries, organization and individuals involved.

Figure 6.2 Understanding the four dimensions of addiction.

if some of these more complex (and expensive) alternatives are in place that their true effectiveness can be judged, compared to methadone: methadone alone does not 'work'.

Implications for public health

The pattern of involvement with illicit drugs can be illustrated as follows: the majority of people have never used illicit drugs; substantial but unclear numbers move into experimentation and more frequent use; at the end of the continuum we find smaller numbers of addicted individuals with an overwhelming involvement in drug use (see Figure 6.3). What could make a difference? Four aims can be identified for a potentially successful drugs strategy.

The first aim is to support and help those in overwhelming involvement back into safer use and, perhaps, abstinence: a process we can term 'care and recovery'. Recovery is a difficult and challenging process. However good

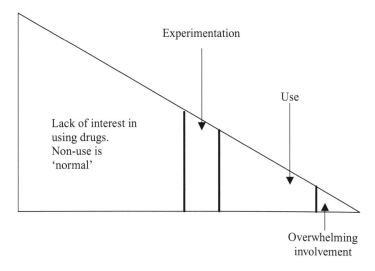

Figure 6.3 Schematic representation of drug use in society.

professional practice may be, in many cases support is simply not provided in the manner that is needed or at the time that it is required. In short, there is a mismatch between the needs of a problem drug user and the ability of agencies, each working from within their own bureaucratic structures, to provide inputs at the right time and with the necessary sensitivity.

The second aim is to stop harm coming to those who are experimenting, using or overwhelmingly involved with drugs. Harm reduction is a key component of an overall strategy but should not be seen as its most important concern. In relation to illegal drugs we have, since the 1980s, pursued a policy aimed more at reducing the harm associated with the use of illegal drugs rather than reducing the scale of such drug use itself. In 1988, the Advisory Council on the Misuse of Drugs' *AIDS and Drugs Misuse Report* included a short sentence which has shaped drug policy and practice in the UK for the last twenty years (Raistrick 1994). The Report stated that: 'The spread of HIV is a greater danger to individual and public health than drug misuse'. The primary object of policy therefore became to reduce drug users' chances of acquiring and spreading HIV infection; in essence, trying to avoid a possible HIV epidemic. From the mid-1990s, when it was evident that HIV was not spreading to anything like the degree that had initially been anticipated (in part because of this policy), the key policy priority shifted towards viewing problem drug use in criminal justice terms with the aim being to reduce the level of drug-related offending. In both cases the focus was on harm to society not the level of drug use or individual recovery.

The third aim is to help individuals to avoid moving down the continuum of non-use to experimentation to use and then overwhelming involvement. The important components of this strategy are to promote non-involvement and to be aware of the pathways into involvement and what works, to prevent progress through a drug or alcohol career. The promotion of non-involvement seems to be dependent on understanding the complex and interacting risk factors (family, community, cultural, economic and structural factors) for involvement, then doing our utmost to foster alternatives and protect those who are at highest risk. So, for example, being brought up in a family that uses drugs, living in a community with low levels of trust and high crime rates, or in a society with steep inequalities, are all seen as risk factors for drug use. Non-involvement might, therefore, be promoted by reversing the adverse consequences of these and many other risk factors. There is also a need to identify key settings and crucial times in the lifecourse where interventions might be most successful. Schools, the most disadvantaged communities, and prisons are obvious examples.

The fourth aim is to shift the distribution of risk of the whole population to the left, which is a whole population strategy (see Figure 6.4). Note how the numbers of people in the categories of concern (overwhelming involvement, use and experimentation) reduce substantially when the whole population shifts its risk to the left (which is analogous to the observations for systolic blood pressure and stroke made in Chapter 2). Another way of thinking about this approach is to use the analogy of an iceberg. Like an iceberg, only a small

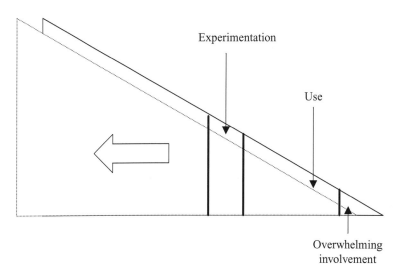

Figure 6.4 Shifting the distribution of risk and use.

proportion of the drugs and alcohol problem is visible and we will never solve the whole problem if we simply chip away at the part that is visible above the surface. Most of the problem is hidden below the surface. Some benefit will be derived from trying to target individuals in this 'hidden problem' group but this is not enough. The only way to shrink the size of the metaphorical iceberg of visible and hidden drug users is to 'raise the temperature of the water': that is, to change the nature of our society so that fewer people develop a problematical relationship with drugs and alcohol.

This is a crucial insight. Much policy attention has focused primarily on *problem* drug or alcohol use, although it is the median level of alcohol consumption in a society that dictates the number of problem drinkers. In other words, it is the *normative attitudes* to drugs that influence the pattern of drug use. Similarly, it is the *overall pattern of inequality* that influences the lives of those living in the most disadvantaged communities. So, such problems are not best conceptualized as confined to a minority. We need to understand the problems of the minority as rather the tip of an iceberg. Since the late 1970s there has been an enlargement of this iceberg in the UK, the surrounding 'water' (the broader social and cultural conditions in which we all live) seems to have been getting colder. That is, there are aspects of modern society that plausibly predispose many of us towards addictive and damaging forms of behaviour, and these seem to be worsening. This prompts the question, what will increase the temperature of the ocean and, therefore, shrink the size of the iceberg?

Conclusions

Obesity and various forms of addiction are not just problems experienced by individuals, requiring individual intervention and treatment. They are examples of the kinds of public health problems that can occur, given the prevailing social, economic and cultural conditions of late modernity. The problem for the public health community is that we often imagine that problems such as obesity and addiction can be solved by tinkering with processes rather than by confronting the root causes: a market economy and a consumer culture. This observation might also provide a useful reminder that many who live in modern society are far from being 'in charge' or in control, whether of our own lives or the direction of our society. Rather, we are all potentially in danger of becoming overwhelmed by our increasing engagement in the values of a market-dominated and growth-driven society – a worldview which is, at the least, damaging to public health and at worst represents a fundamental threat. Nevertheless, the public health problems addressed in this chapter, though serious and worsening, do not yet affect entire populations. The final chapter in this section of the book turns to a number of public health challenges which do that and more: the emergence of a set of interconnected problems which undermine not just human health and well-being, but the sustainability of human society itself.

References

Alexander, B.K. (2008) *The Globalisation of Addictions*. Oxford: Oxford University Press.

Bobak, M. and Marmot, M. (1994) *The East–West health divide and potential explanations*. Paper presented to the European Health Policy Conference: Opportunities for the Future, Copenhagen, 5–9 December.

Braet, C., Mervielde, I. and Vandereycken, W. (1997) Psychological aspects of childhood obesity: a controlled study in a clinical and non-clinical sample. *Journal of Paediatric Psychology*, 22(1): 59–71.

Centers for Disease Control and Prevention (2010) *Obesity at a Glance 2010: Halting the Epidemic by Making Health Easier*. Atlanta: National Center for Chronic Disease Prevention and Health Promotion.

Counihan, C. (1999) *The Anthropology of Food and Body: Gender, Meaning and Power*. New York: Routledge.

Durkheim, E. (1897/1952) *Suicide: a Study in Sociology*. London: Routledge and Kegan Paul.

Foresight Report (2007) *Tackling Obesity – Future Choices: Project Report*. London: Government Office for Science.

Homer-Dixon, T. (2000) *The Ingenuity Gap: Facing the Economic, Environmental, and Other Challenges of an Increasingly Complex and Unpredictable Future*. London: Jonathan Cape.

Jernigan, D.H., Monteiro, M., Room, R. and Saxena, S. (2000) Towards a global alcohol policy: alcohol, public health and the role of WHO. *Bulletin of the World Health Organization*, 78: 491–9.

McKee, M. and Leon, D.A. (2005) Social transition and substance abuse. *Addiction*, 100: 1205–9.

Mintz, S.W. and Du Bois, C.M. (2002) The anthropology of food and eating. *Annual Review of Anthropology*, 31: 99–119.

NHS Information Centre: Lifestyle Statistics (2010) *Statistics on Physical Activity, Obesity and Diet: England 2010*. London: NHS Health and Social Care Information Centre.

Nishida, C., Uauy, R., Kumanyika, S. and Shetty, P. (2002) The Joint WHO/FAO Expert Consultation on diet, nutrition and the prevention of chronic diseases: process, product and policy implications. *Public Health Nutrition*, 7(1A): 245–50.

Popkin, B. (2009) *The World is Fat: The Fads, Trends, Policies and Products that are Fattening the Human Race*. New York: Penguin.

Raistrick, D.S. (1994) Report of Advisory Council on the Misuse of Drugs: AIDS and drug misuse update (editorial). *Addiction*, 89: 1211–13.

Sassi, F., Devaux, M., Cecchini, M. and Rusticelli, E. (2009) *The Obesity Epidemic: Analysis of Past and Projected Future Trends in Selected OECD Countries*. OECD Health Working Papers, No. 45. OECD Publishing

Seidell, J.C. and Flegal, K.M. (1997) Assessing obesity: classification and epidemiology. *British Medical Bulletin*, 53(2): 238–52.

Sheron, N., Harrkey, C. and Gilmore, I. (2011) Projections of alcohol deaths – a wake-up call. *Lancet*, 377: 1297–9.

United Nations Office on Drugs and Crime (2010) *World Drug Report – Global Illicit Drug Trends*. Vienna: United Nations Office on Drugs and Crime.

West, R. (1997) Addiction, ethics and public policy. *Addiction*, 92: 1061–70.

Wilkinson, R.G. (1996) *Unhealthy Societies: The Afflictions of Inequality*. London: Routledge.

Wilkinson, R.G. and Pickett, K.E. (2006) Income inequality and population health: a review and explanation of the evidence. *Social Science and Medicine*, 62: 1768–84.

Wilkinson, R. and Pickett, K. (2009) *The Spirit Level: Why More Equal Societies Almost Always Do Better*. London: Allen Lane.

World Health Organization (1986) *Ottawa Charter for Health Promotion*. Geneva: World Health Organization.

World Health Organization (2011) Health and Statistics Information System: global burden of disease. http://www.who.int/healthinfo/global _burden_disease/estimates_country/en/index.html. (accessed February 2011).

Wright, C.M., Parker, L., Lamont, D. and Craft, A.W. (2001) Implications of childhood obesity for adult health: findings from thousand families cohort study. *British Medical Journal*, 323(1): 1280–4.

7 Population growth and ageing

Introduction

One of the key messages of this chapter is that public health requires a better understanding of the implications of emerging and future demographic change for the longer-term sustainability of global human society (Brown and Kane 1995; Barber 2001). The latter issue is the specific focus of the next chapter, where other factors which impact on sustainability are reviewed from a public health perspective. In the context of this chapter, some grasp of demographic change over the course of human history is helpful. We know that population growth was very slow for many millennia but is now accelerating in many parts of the world (Gallant 1990). It took, for example, 2 million years for the global human population to reach a billion people but only 130 years to add the second billion. It then took 30 years to add the third billion people, 15 years to add the fourth, and only 12 years to add the fifth. At the current rate of growth, it now takes about ten months to add 75 million people to the global population (which is the number of people killed by bubonic plague over the centuries), or 1.7 years to add 165 million (which is the number of people killed in wars during the past 200 years). The global population of 7 billion in 2011 is projected to increase to at least 9.3 billion by the year 2050 (United Nations Department of Economic and Social Affairs 2004). What will this mean for human society, in the context of a planet with finite resources? This is an important question for the public health community.

The chapter briefly describes global patterns of population growth and decline. Such patterns are determined by three factors: births, deaths and migration. The chapter then explains the relationship between population growth and fertility rates. It describes the five stages of the demographic transition that most nations are predicted to pass through at various points in their economic development. The chapter then describes the problem, for some affluent nations, of population replacement levels and the dependency ratio. The chapter outlines the concept of the earth's 'carrying capacity' in terms of humanity's resource demands and their relationship to population growth. It describes how, in comparatively recent times, such growth was prompted by two unique and unrepeatable events in human history. The chapter concludes by highlighting the implications for the healthy ageing of populations, which is an important public health goal.

Population growth and decline

Each region of the globe has seen great reductions in population growth rate in recent decades, though these remain above two per cent in some countries of the Middle East and sub-Saharan Africa and in areas of South Asia, Southeast Asia, and Latin America (United Nations Department of Economic and Social Affairs 2004). The relationship between population growth rates and the time it takes to double the population is simple: it is called the rule of 70. The doubling time is 70 divided by the annual growth rate. So, countries in sub-Saharan Africa with growth rates of two per cent will double their populations in 35 years. This means that those countries will need to build twice the number of schools, hospitals and houses and create twice as many jobs as they have at present, in just over three decades – a daunting challenge for even the most affluent nation (Institut Nationale d'Etudies Demographique 1988).

Globally, the growth rate of the human population peaked in 1963 at 2.20 per cent per annum: since then, it has been declining. In 2009, the estimated annual growth rate was 1.1 per cent. The actual annual growth in the number of humans fell from a peak of 88 million per year in 1989, to a low of 73.9 million in 2003, after which it rose again to 75.2 million in 2006. In 2009 the human population increased by 74.6 million but this annual growth total is projected to fall steadily to about 41 million per year in 2050, at which time the population will have increased to a total of around 9.2 billion. During the period up to 2050 the population of the industrialized world will probably remain largely static while the population of developing countries will increase from about 5.3 billion to almost 8 billion (United Nations Department of Economic and Social Affairs 2004). Current predictions are that the globe's population will eventually peak in 2070 and then slowly decline. How the future for humankind turns out will depend on the speed with which the whole world's population growth figure declines, as even a few more years of modest growth in an already large number will add considerably to the eventual peak figure (Lutz et al. 2004).

Population fertility rates

Two types of fertility rates affect a country's population size and growth rate. The replacement-level fertility is the number of children a couple must have, to replace them. This figure is always higher than 2 (examples include 2.1 children for an industrialized country and 2.5 children for a less developed country) because some female children die before reaching their reproductive years. A more useful measure is the total fertility rate (TFR), which is an estimate of the average number of children born to a woman during her reproductive years (i.e. ages 15–44). This is an artificial construct based on population-based age-specific rates. A simpler way of thinking about the TFR is as the average number of children a woman will bear. A key question, therefore, is what factors affect birth rates. In the example of the UK's transition, the main factors included: average level of education and affluence; the role of children as part of the family labour force; urbanization (which reduces family size); costs of raising children; education and employment opportunities for women; average age at marriage; infant mortality rates; availability of birth control; and religious and cultural norms.

During the twentieth century the global population mushroomed but towards the end of the century the rate of growth declined. During the 1970s women around the world had six children on average. That figure has since declined: in some countries it is below replacement level (i.e. 2.1 children). In Italy it has fallen to 1.3 and the general trend in Europe is for lowering fertility rates. Japan has very similar rates and in Asia as a whole the fertility rate is down from 2.4 in 1970 to 1.5 today. Developed parts of East Asia in particular have plummeted rapidly to low levels of fertility which took Europe decades to attain. China's fertility rate has declined from 6.06 to 1.8 children, and is still declining. Conversely, the poorest Asian countries still have high fertility; Afghanistan, for example, has a fertility rate of 7.1.

However, even in those countries where the growth rate is slowing, fertility rates remain well above replacement levels (a concept which is explained below). Also, countries that now show modest population growth still add large numbers to the global population each year simply because of the size of their populations. For example, India's modest 1.4 per cent annual rate adds 26 million people to the census each year. This momentum of growth comes from the size of the population and its young age structure as well as its fertility rate. In addition, while life expectancy is still short compared with many industrialized nations, people in most developing nations are now beginning to live longer, which is a welcome development (Freedman 2008).

The demographic transition

The demographic transition is the term used to describe the move from high birth and death rates and low life expectancy to low birth and low death rates and high life expectancy (Caldwell et al. 2006). In almost all cases, this type of demographic transition accompanies a move from a pre-industrial to an

Table 7.1 Summary of the demographic transition

Before the demographic transition	After the demographic transition
Birth rates high	Birth rates low
Death rates high	Death rates low
Life expectancy low	Life expectancy high
Population smaller	Population larger
Population growth high	Population growth low or declining

industrialized economy. The transition involves five stages (summarized in Table 7.1):

1   Stage one (pre-industrial society) is characterized by a balance between birth rates and death rates. Birth and death rates are very high and their approximate balance results in very slow population growth.
2   In stage two, population growth begins solely due to a decrease in death rates, while birth rates stay high (i.e. there are fewer deaths rather than more births). More children enter the reproductive cycle of their lives while still maintaining the high fertility rates of their parents. This causes the bottom of the age pyramid to widen, accelerating population growth.
3   In stage 3, the population moves towards stability and population growth levels off through a decline in the birth rate.
4   Stage four is characterized by stability: there are both low birth rates and low death rates.
5   Stage five is characterized by the shift to a post-industrial, service-led economy. In this stage, birth rates are lower than death rates, leading to a decline in population levels.

The conventional wisdom about demographic transition (the five stages set out above) is that when people are poor they have many children. In simple terms, if half of your children die before adulthood then you need to have more, in order to ensure there is someone to look after you in old age. As people get richer, family size starts to drop: the health of children improves; girls go to school and get jobs, marry later and have children later. However, there are exceptions to this generalized pattern. Korea was not rich when fertility declined. Conversely, the Gulf States are rich but have high fertility. In short, cultural and other factors (such as religious beliefs) are also important. The world's highest fertility rates are to be found in the most religious countries, with the exception of the very low fertility rates found in Catholic southern Europe.

Population movement and migration

Alongside the rapid global growth in population, other associated dynamics are also playing out. When the UK went through its demographic transition, many of its growing population migrated to North America, Australia, New Zealand and parts of Africa. Today's migrants, like those of the late nineteenth and early twentieth centuries, are following the money. The search for new economic opportunities is driving a massive migration in the global population from south to north and east to west. Between 1970 and 2000 the international migrant population doubled from 82 million to 175 million. Currently, one out of every thirty-five human beings in the world is an international migrant. These trends are almost certain to continue and accelerate. In most developing nations there is also a continuing drift towards urban living. For the first time in their history, the majority of humans live in cities (Global Urban Observatory and Statistics Unit 2005). One consequence is that the number of 'megacities' – those with populations over 10 million – continues to grow rapidly (Homer-Dixon 2006). This growth is particularly rapid in developing countries where people migrate to cities out of economic necessity, unable to find sustaining livelihoods in rural areas as the productivity of the land is compromised by human demands, and the prices paid for food do not adequately reflect its value. Forty-three per cent of the urban population of poor countries now live in slums (Homer-Dixon 2006), with obvious negative consequences for their health. The pressure on population and resources in poorer countries is already intense and will increase over time.

Population replacement levels and the dependency ratio

In most Western European countries birth rates are now below replacement levels and the population is ageing significantly. Nevertheless, the population in most of these European countries is still growing, largely because of migration. Countries that have low birth rates and high life expectancies express concerns about their *dependency ratio*: that is, the proportion of the population who are dependent because they are young, retired, unemployed, disabled or sick compared to those who are in paid employment. The conventional wisdom is that migrant workers can help alleviate these pressures. Migrants make many contributions to their host nation for all sorts of reasons but rich countries that encourage migration simply because of their own demographic and economic concerns ignore two important considerations:

- First, the globe may already be past its carrying capacity and densely populated nations like the UK only maintain their populations by exploiting large areas of other countries for resources, agriculture and manufacture, with consequences for the longer term health and well-being of people living in the exploited regions.
- Second, the whole world is moving rapidly to a point where all populations will be relatively old but stable, so the dependency ratio problem cannot be solved by migration.

Population growth and interacting human systems

Population growth *per se* is not a problem (Freedman 2008). However, when combined with several other aspects of human systems and their interaction with each other and the biosphere, the result is a significant public health challenge. For example, how to feed the world's (present) seven billion and (future) ten billion people (Evans 1998). According to the world food programme, the total number of malnourished people fell from 959 million to 791 million during the period 1990–1997. This decline was mainly due to improved nutrition in India and China as these countries developed. The number of malnourished people started to grow again by the end of the decade and by 2001–2003, the number of chronically hungry in the world stood at 854 million. Since then, the situation has not improved and periodic hikes in food prices have caused increasing hardship and political unrest. This puts hunger among the top threats to health worldwide (Freedman 1998).

According to the US Agency for International Development, hunger leading to malnutrition accounted for about 53 per cent of preschool deaths in the world in 2005. Each year, malnutrition kills 6 million children; that is, one every five seconds. It is tempting to suggest that the solution to this problem is to grow more food. However, we live in a world where there are more obese people than malnourished or hungry people. This suggests that the overall volume of food supply is not the only or perhaps even the main problem. Most of the 'grow more' solutions are also affected by the impacts of other challenges that we now face. For example, chemical fertilizers, the backbone of the green revolution since the 1960s, are intimately linked to the price of oil, which is becoming more unstable than in the past. Most food ecologies will be affected by climate change. Valuable agricultural land, which could be used for food, is passing over to the growing of bio-fuels. As forests are cleared for planting, rich topsoil is washed away. In any case, it is most likely that there has been enough food in the world to feed everyone since 1945, yet 850 million go hungry every day. So, population growth interacts with issues like climate change, economic development policy, increasing natural resource use and environmental depletion, the industrialized production of food, and the global economic politics of food production and distribution.

Population growth and global carrying capacity

What seems clear is that the whole world is in this together. Population growth and numbers matter but cannot be dissociated from resources and consumption (McMichael 2001). In this context, the world's 'carrying capacity' is the maximum population that can be permanently supported. Any land area of the globe has a finite carrying capacity for humans and the globe as a whole has a finite carrying capacity (Brown and Kane 1995). This issue is important at two levels:

- At a local level, human numbers have frequently exceeded carrying capacity and this has led to wars. For example, it has been argued that the killing of one ethnic group by another on the scale witnessed in Rwanda was a war of carrying capacity and reflected a growing shortage of agricultural land in that fertile but densely populated country.
- At a planetary level, many expert commentators argue that the world's population, with its current technologies and consumption patterns, has already exceeded the planet's carrying capacity.

Although carrying capacity is finite, it is not fixed. Two comparatively recent but unique events in human history changed the earth's carrying capacity. The first was the discovery and exploitation, from the fifteenth century onwards, of the vast landmass of the 'New World' of North and South America. The second was the discovery of fossil fuels.

When Europeans first arrived in the 'New World' they perceived it as largely empty. It was sparsely populated with indigenous tribes which pursued a mainly hunter-gatherer way of life mixed with some agrarian activity. These indigenous peoples needed the full land area for their way of life. The European settlers and colonists came from a continent that had a relatively advanced agriculture. A farmer with the cumulated knowledge of many generations of farming, a metal plough and a draft animal could grow enough food for his family, his animals and have some left over. This surplus meant that a larger proportion of the population could engage in activities beyond subsistence farming. Europeans had also developed firearms, which made hunting for animals much easier. In the sixteen generations following the development of hand-held firearms the average rate of population increase became higher than at any previous time of human history. Europe was beginning to reach its carrying capacity when the New World was opened up as a destination for emigration and exploitation.

From the perspective of the indigenous populations of America, the settlers were competing for the available land. Firearms gave the settlers the advantage but did not enlarge the planet: they merely enlarged the carrying capacity of the world by making more land available for settlement and exploitation. In 1492 when the Americas were first 'discovered' there were roughly 24 acres of Europe for each European. Once Europeans colonized the new lands, that ratio increased to 120 acres per European. This created a new spirit of abundance and one of the results was that, between 1650 and 1850, the global human population doubled. With this level of population growth, even within North America the ratio of land to people fell by 1850 to 11 acres per person. This was less than half the European ratio that had caused profound population pressures at the time Columbus set sail, in 1492.

Carrying capacity was changed again by the discovery and use of fossil fuels as part of the industrial revolution. The industrial revolution, with its four waves of health improvement, decreased death rates and extended life expectancy in a remarkable manner. Industrialization made available the accumulated solar energy of many millennia, stored in fossil fuels such as oil and natural gas. It increased the proportion of the earth's surface that could be exploited by humans and massively increased our capacity to grow and move food. By drawing on energy stores from the earth's deep geological past, industrialization moved at a pace fast enough to create wealth that led to an increase in human numbers and a rise in per capita wealth. One side effect of this process is that some of the most densely populated spots on earth, like London, New York, Hong Kong and Tokyo, are among the most prosperous, healthy and well nourished. People in these global centres of wealth creation have in recent years talked about the evolution of a 'weightless' economy that relies on ideas and not materials to create wealth. Yet the resource upon which this exponential rise in human numbers and prosperity has been based is finite, drawn from the past, arguably stolen from the future and potentially toxic (in terms of climate change) to the planet.

The concept of an 'ecological footprint' illustrates the limits of the planet's carrying capacity by comparing human demands on nature with the biosphere's ability to regenerate resources and provide services. The acreage of land and sea needed to fully sustain a given population is calculated, including land for food and other resources as well to absorb pollutants produced by that population. In this way it is possible to calculate the footprint of a city, a country or the whole world's population. This work demonstrates why densely populated cities can be incredibly wealthy: they have a massive ecological footprint and could not survive without access through trade to vast tracts of land beyond their borders.

There is a growing literature that highlights the conclusion that we may already have gone beyond the human carrying capacity of the environment by continuing with behaviours that are no longer appropriate for present circumstances. This suggests that the whole world needs a stable or slowly declining population which operates at a sustainable level of consumption. If that happens, the whole globe will be in stage four or five of the demographic transition, which means that the whole world will have the age profile currently found in Europe, North America and Japan. That makes the population dynamics of ageing a vitally important issue for public health and human development.

Population ageing and dependency

Low fertility rates in rich countries may lead to rapid population ageing. If Europe continues at a replacement level of 1.5 children, the population will halve in 65 years. The European Union has an ageing community but countries within the Union are ageing at different rates. Ireland has the youngest population; Sweden has the oldest, followed by Germany, France and the UK. At the turn of the twentieth century, one fifth of the population was aged over 60 years but by 2020 this group will constitute one quarter. In policy terms, the rise of the proportion of the population over 80 years of age is probably of greater significance. Women predominate in all the higher ranges of the age pyramid (see Figure 7.1).

As Figure 7.1 shows, using Scotland as an example of demographic change in the UK, the 'baby boomers' (those born between 1945 and 1956) are a very large post-Second World War age cohort. This group is now moving into old age and will create a large and significant increase in the older population, not only in absolute numbers but also in relation to the numbers of people of working age. The ageing of society has implications for the so-called 'old-age dependency ratio': the ratio of individuals aged 65 and over to the size of the economically active segment of the population. In the UK, for every 100 people aged 15–64, the number of people aged 65 and over will grow from just less than 18 per cent in 1960 to a predicted 29.7 per cent in 2025. It is widely assumed that this shift in the balance of older and working age people in the population will damage the economy and create serious problems for health and social care services (Pol and Thomas 2001). Not only is it predicted that there will be an insufficient number of taxpayers to pay for the costs of the NHS (16- to 44-year-olds cost £350 a head in NHS spending whereas the comparable figure for the retired is £2,700), but there will not be sufficient numbers of young people to work as health and social care professionals.

The developing world is also ageing rapidly. Of the eleven largest elderly populations in the world, eight are found within the developing world (China, India, Brazil, Indonesia, Pakistan, Mexico, Bangladesh and Nigeria). With few exceptions, the elderly are now the fastest growing segment in the developing world (Pol and Thomas 2001; United Nations Population Division 2002). The

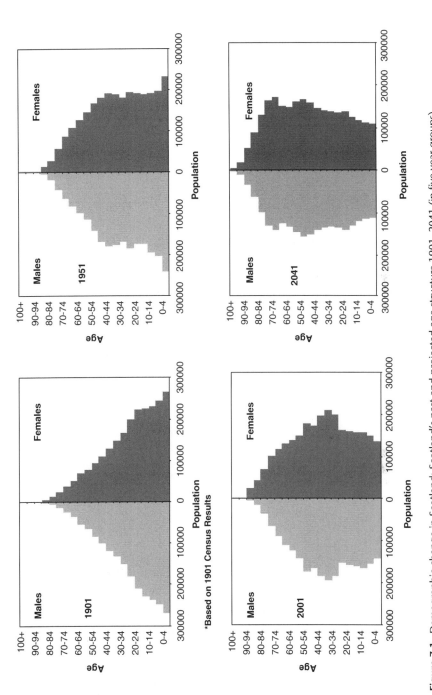

Figure 7.1 Demographic change in Scotland: Scotland's past and projected age structure 1901–2041 (in five year groups).
Source: GROS 1901 census, 1951 and 2001 mid-year estimates and 2004 based projections

pace of demographic transition varies from country to country. It took, for instance, 115 years (1865–1980) for the proportion of older people in France to increase from 7 per cent to 14 per cent. The equivalent time for the same doubling to happen in China is expected to be 27 years (2000–2027). The Chinese population will have far less time to change and adapt services and their economy.

Age and health

As we age the risk of disease and death increases. The reason for this is that ageing leads to a progressive, generalized impairment of function resulting in a loss of adaptive response. A wide range of physiological functions decline with age: examples include the efficiency of lung function, circulation, muscles and nerves. There would seem to be a genetic element to this process of decline but it is also influenced by factors like environment, lifestyle and nutrition. Under certain influences this decline can accelerate but attention to behaviour and environment can significantly slow the decline. For example, those who do not use their large muscle groups will lose strength. Sometimes the level of decline is such that we define it as pathological. For example, an individual who smokes and eats a high fat diet may experience changes that reduce coronary blood flow and lead to ischaemic heart disease. The key point is that there is a slow decline in a wide range of physiological functions with age but that the rate of decline is amenable to a large variety of environmental and behavioural interventions. Other factors include being mentally as well as physically active, feeling able to contribute to society, and having good relationships with others.

External assaults that become more common with ageing include accidents, trauma, infections and carcinogens. The environment in which we live influences the frequency and scale of such assaults. Also, our ability to withstand, for example, infection or trauma depends on the reserve capacity of our physiological systems: pneumonia in a young healthy person with lungs that have a large reserve capacity is much less likely to be fatal than the same infection in an older person with a lifelong history of smoking. This analysis suggests that healthy ageing means minimizing physiological decline (in parallel across the major body systems) and external assaults like trauma, infection and carcinogens. The term 'compression of morbidity' describes a scenario where increasing proportions of the population will achieve these twin aims and live a long, healthy life in which death will be preceded by a very short period of ill health (morbidity). This scenario is based on a few key assumptions.

First, that the human lifespan is not endlessly elastic: while increasingly large proportions of the population will achieve old age, the lifespan will not be pushed much higher. Second, if increasingly large proportions of the population can achieve slow and parallel physiological decline and a mini-mization of external assaults, we will achieve healthy ageing for the majority of people. An alternative theory is that we will see an extension to the period of ill health and poor functioning at the end of life: an extension, rather than compression, of morbidity. Two mechanisms will drive this. The first is that the age of onset of poor function or disease will remain unchanged because influences like smoking and poor diet will give rise to, for example, coronary heart disease, diabetes or obstructive airways disease during mid-life. The second is that medical and environmental interventions will allow people to survive to an older age, the consequence of which will be increased longevity but with an extended period of morbidity.

Conclusion

The growing global population is an important public health challenge we face, the significance of which goes beyond sheer numbers of people. In the absence of some truly catastrophic event that decimates existing populations, the demographic transition appears to be an inevitable – and in many ways desirable – global phenomenon. If populations succeed in moving through the type of economic and social development experienced by Europe since the 1850s, demographic transition is the likely outcome. If the whole world moves through the demographic transition the global population will stabilize at between nine and ten billion people. This may or may not be sustainable, depending on the pressures so large a population places on the world's nat-ural resources. What is certain is that such numbers cannot be sustained at the levels of consumption currently found in affluent/Western-type societies. It therefore seems likely that the issue of a planned population decline may return to the international development agenda (Brown et al. 2000). The alter-native to population stability/decline is runaway population growth, as even very modest global rates of growth add very large numbers as the total pop-ulation size increases. The danger is that runaway growth would be followed by population collapse.

The corollary of the demographic transition will be a globally stable pop-ulation with a median age in the mid-50s: as Figure 7.1 above illustrates, the population 'pyramid' will come to look more like a rectangle. The ageing of the global population will place strains on services and change the way in which we live (older retirement age in developed societies is an obvious example). This means that the need to compress morbidity and create con-ditions in which most people can achieve a healthy old age will become one of the greatest priorities for public health during this century. However, to achieve the best case scenario for a healthy ageing population, at least three conditions will have to be met. First, the whole world will have to adapt to a stable but relatively older population structure. Second, the poorest countries of the world will require adequate resources to ensure their appropriate and adequate economic development. Third, global resource utilization should be more equitable and will have to become sustainable. It is to this key issue of sustainability that we turn in the next chapter.

References

Barber, N. (2001) *Coping with Population Growth (the Environmental Challenge)*. London: Raintree.

Brown, L. and Kane, L. (1995) *Full House: Reassessing the Earth's Population Carrying Capacity*. London: Earthscan.

Brown, L.R., Gardner, G. and Halweil, B. (2000) *Beyond Malthus: Nineteen Dimensions of the Population Challenge*. London: Earthscan.

Caldwell, J.C., Cardwell, B.K., Caldwell, P., McDonald, P.F. and Schindlmayr, T. (2006) *Demographic Transition Theory*. Dordrecht: Springer.

Evans, L.T. (1998) *Feeding the Ten Billions: Plants and Population Growth*. Cambridge: Cambridge University Press.

Freedman, R. (ed.) (2008) *Population Growth: The Vital Revolution*. Piscataway: Aldine Transactions.

Gallant, R.A. (1990) *Peopling of Planet Earth: Human Population Growth Through the Ages*. Englewood Cliffs: Prentice-Hall.

Global Urban Observatory and Statistics Unit (2005) Global Trends 2005. http://www.unhabitat.org/habrdd/global.html (accessed 16 September 2011).

Homer-Dixon, T. (2006) *The Upside of Down: Catastrophe, Creativity and the Renewal of Civilisation*. London: Souvenir Press.

Institut National d'Etudies Demographiques (1988) *Consequences of Rapid Population Growth in Developing Countries*. New York: Taylor & Francis.

Lutz, W., Sanderson, W. and Scherbov, S. (2004) *End of World Population Growth in 21st Century: New Challenges for Human Capital Formation and Sustainable Development*. London: Earthscan.

McMichael, A.J. (2001) *Human Frontiers, Environments and Disease*. Cambridge: Cambridge University Press.

Pol, L.G. and Thomas, R.K. (2001) *The Demography of Health and Health Care (The Plenum Series on Demographic Methods and Population Analysis)*, 2nd edn. New York: Kluwer Academic Publishers.

United Nations Department of Economic and Social Affairs (UNDESA) (2004) *World Population to 2300*. New York: United Nations.

United Nations Population Division (2002) World population prospects: the 2002 revision. http://www.un.org/esa/population/publications/wpp2002/WPP2002-HIGHLIGHTSrev1.PDF

8 Public health and the challenge of sustainability

Introduction

The previous chapter focused on one of the most important factors affecting the longer term sustainability of human society: demographic change. This chapter moves on to look at the emergence of broader global problems that threaten to destabilize some of the Earth's systems, disrupt life in many societies, and threaten the existence of many species of plant and animal life (Brown 1996; Kunstler 2005). In particular, we point to the connection between climate change, 'peak oil', and the looming collision between our environment and our economy. The public health community needs to understand the interactions and synergies between these phenomena. The significant reduction in life expectancy that accompanied the end of Soviet communism in the late twentieth century is an example of a public health calamity caused by dramatic social, political and economic upheaval. Yet the health and well-being threats implicit in climate change and other ecological problems discussed in this chapter are potentially far more profound. Much excellent public health literature focuses on pathways from ecological collapse to human disease via the physical and biological environment (e.g. Haines et al. 2006, 2007; McMichael et al. 2006; Costello et al. 2009). However, many societies (including our own) face the looming prospect of ecological collapse that will lead to economic collapse, which will be accompanied by social collapse, on a scale that might make the public health problems of the former Soviet bloc seem small by comparison.

We know that the Earth is a dynamic and changing system: scientific study of its past shows considerable shifts in atmosphere, temperature, ice cover, sea levels and more. We also know that past human civilizations have been affected considerably by such changes and that our growing and globalized civilization is now facing a threat to its survival (Mackenbach 2007; Smith et al. 2009; Davis et al. 2010). Some of the most significant challenges facing everyone in the modern world are anthropogenic climate change and environmental depletion. To these we also need to add exponential economic growth and 'peak oil' (Roberts 2005; Stiglitz 2010). A key point for the public health community is that this set of threats to the sustainability of human and many other forms of life on Earth have combined to create conditions of planetary overload. The best-publicized ecological problem is probably climate change but even if that problem were to disappear tomorrow, threats to the sustainability of our civilization from the other sources could be as great. A second key point is that interactions and synergies exist between this set of sustainability threats, which also have to be understood in the context of the exponential population growth discussed in Chapter 7. Together, they represent a concatenation of troubles that challenge human ingenuity (Homer-Dixon 2000). These – and their public health implications – are briefly described in the sections below.

Climate change

Climate change is both a major threat to public health worldwide and an additional source of widening inequalities between rich and poor (Wilkinson et al. 2007). Some description of the mechanics of the processes involved in climate change is needed here. Energy which reaches the Earth in the form of solar radiation warms our planet while energy leaving as invisible infrared radiation cools it. The Earth's temperature results from the balance between these two. A change in that balance has resulted in the world's average surface temperature increasing by approximately 0.6°C during the twentieth century (approximately two-thirds of that warming since 1975). Climatologists judge most of that recent increase is due to human influence and forecast further warming during the twenty-first century, along with changes in precipitation and climatic variability. World temperatures now exceed the upper limit of natural (historical) variability and the Intergovernmental Panel on Climate Change (2007) estimates that a doubling of carbon dioxide (CO_2) concentration in the Earth's atmosphere in the current century will heat the planet's surface by between 2°C and 4.5°C, with an increase of 3°C being the most likely (Lynas 2008).

A second major greenhouse gas is methane. Major human-produced sources of methane in the atmosphere include energy production, emissions from livestock, landfills, biomass burning and waste treatment (McMichael et al. 2007). There are also huge reserves of natural methane currently trapped and frozen as methane hydrate at the bottom of the ocean, the steppes of Russia, the arctic permafrost and the Siberian peat bogs. It is thought that, in the future, thawing of this ice due to global warming could release large quantities of methane which in turn will cause a further temperature rise. The predicted increase of atmospheric methane could cause an average global temperature increase of 5°C, in addition to the 2–3°C increase which will occur even if there is no drop in CO_2 emissions. This is why many climate scientists argue that the overall global temperature rise must be kept below 2°C, the tipping point at which methane release could lead to positive feedback and runaway climate change.

Other mechanisms could also lead to positive feedback loops being established once the temperature rise goes much above 2°C. Livestock, for example, generate 18 per cent of human activity related greenhouse gases (McMichael et al. 2007). While cattle produce nine per cent of human related carbon dioxide, they are responsible for 65 per cent of the more potent greenhouse gas nitrous oxide and 37 per cent of all human induced methane. As countries in the developing world become wealthier, they consume more meat, for which more cattle are required: this is an example of how greenhouse gases will probably increase. Current concentrations of greenhouse gases are unprecedented in human history, and are accompanied by the progressive transformation of landscapes, degradation of ecosystems, acidification of the oceans, and the extinction of species, with incalculable effects (UNEP 2009).

We can already see the impacts of global warming in, for example, retreating glaciers, reduced polar ice cover and melting permafrost. These great sheets of ice are not susceptible to the warm weather of a single warm summer but show longer trends in heating and cooling. This also has great significance for river flow. For example, something approaching 80 per cent of the dry season flow of the Indo-Gangetic plain comes from the previous season's snow fall in the high ranges of Ladakh. Without this snow, the dry season flow of India's great rivers will be about 20 per cent of the current level. Similar processes are occurring in many other river systems, with devastating impacts on irrigation and agriculture, and thus food as well as water supply. The global climate will also be 'livelier', with faster, wetter storms in northern latitudes, and more severe flooding worldwide. It is predicted that by the 2040s the high temperatures ('heat wave') which caused excess deaths in Europe in 2003 will look normal; by the 2060s they will look cool. Changes in climate already contribute to the burden of disease on a global scale and this contribution is expected to rise sharply. Changes in the geographical areas inhabited by vector borne diseases can potentially affect the lives of billions. Other global problems which can affect public health include food and water shortages. In these circumstances, our species is faced with an adaptive imperative: if current temperature trends continue, we are most likely past the point of being able to avoid warming altogether.

Such is the extent and rapidity of change that modern societies are considered instrumental in a new phase of Earth's evolution: the Anthropocene Age. While climate science is a science of uncertainty, recent observations have continually exceeded worst-case scenarios, and evidence has proved robust in the face of intense scrutiny. Risks of non-linear change cannot be dismissed: past episodes of rapid increases in atmospheric carbon have been associated with temperature rises of 5–8°C and abrupt changes in climate, land and water resources. The broad public health implication is that societies would face major social breakdown, loss of life and potential large-scale conflict due to collapsing socio-technical infrastructures and lack of shelter, food and water (Diamond 2005; Haines et al. 2006; Human Development Report 2007/2008; Intergovernmental Panel on Climate Change 2007; Stern 2007; UNEP 2009).

Peak oil

Since the early 1900s, much development has been based on the availability of cheap oil. This includes the production of fertilizers which support intensive farming techniques; the 'just-in-time' retail trade supported by a massive truck fleet; and the out-of-town shopping centres and suburbia developed without need for public transport. Almost every aspect of the society in which we live (including our health service) is currently dependent either directly or indirectly on the availability of cheap oil. It is now known that the peak of oil discovery was reached in the late 1970s. While new fields are still being discovered (largely in the form of tar sands and oil shale) the rate of discovery has been diminishing for decades. Since that time we have been using three barrels of oil for every new one discovered.

Experts within (and outside) the oil industry debate the question of whether we have already reached the second 'peak oil' stage first proposed by geologist M. Hubbert (1945). This is the peak in oil production, which will occur once half the world's oil has been extracted: it then becomes increasingly difficult and expensive to extract the remaining reserve and there will be less oil to go around. Add to this unfolding scenario the increasing internal use of oil by oil producers like Mexico and Nigeria, and the mounting demand from the rapidly industrializing nations such as China, India, Brazil and Indonesia, and it becomes clear that we are moving into uncharted territory with worrying potential for global conflict.

The confident prediction is that the oil price increases that we have seen in recent years will not only be sustained but will accelerate in the future. The price of oil may fluctuate in the short term but the longer term trend will be an inexorable increase. There are historical precedents that should raise concerns. In 1973, following the Yom Kippur war, the first OPEC production restriction of under 10 per cent resulted in a greater than threefold increase in the price of oil. As a result of the oil price rise there was a massive increase in government debt in countries around the world. The increase in price and restrictions on oil production during the 1970s also led to deindustrialization in Europe, as the competitive advantage of oil-importing countries vanished. The scale of this historical price rise was tempered by an increase in exploration and oil discovery (including the UK's North Sea oil field) that increased the supply of oil. The outcome of a peak oil scenario will be different because there will be no new reserves to exploit.

Crucial to the understanding of a peak in production is the finite and concentrated nature of fossil fuels. Oil, gas and other fossil fuels were formed over a period of millions of years from crushed micro-organisms and can essentially be thought of as concentrated solar energy stored in the Earth's crust. Because of the extended period of time necessary to produce this resource, it can be thought of as a one-off and finite endowment. It is unlikely that biofuels will be able to fill the energy gap since they derive their energy from a single year of solar energy, and so could provide only a fraction of the energy contained within fossil fuels (even if bio-fuel farming covered all of the cultivable land on the globe). The diminishing returns from oil exploration and discovery should also be considered. When oil was first drilled it was close to the surface, under high pressure, and of good quality. Since then the most profitable sources have been used up, leaving only the more difficult, expensive and lower quality sources. It is also worth noting that the 'peak oil' phenomenon is not restricted to crude oil but includes natural gas, many minerals and substrates such as uranium. For finite resources such as these, the debate should centre on questions of when and how quickly the decline will happen, not if.

The peak oil phenomenon has worrying implications for global inequalities and international relations (Homer-Dixon 2000; Simms et al. 2004; Haines et al. 2006). There is a widespread belief that wars for oil resources are already underway, prior to the production peak. Under a peak oil scenario the imperative for oil resources is likely to be even greater, particularly in oil-dependent countries such as the United States and China. The impact that this may have on international relations (particularly with the Middle East) and the potential for war is not insignificant. Public health professionals will also be concerned about the impact of rising oil prices on the economy. Unemployment, insecure employment, poverty, fuel poverty, cutbacks in public services and many more adverse effects could follow a recession induced by rising oil prices. There is clear evidence that economic shocks destroy health, as was seen in the health trends of the population in the former Soviet Union, the depression in the United States during the 1920s, and with Scottish deindustrialization in the 1970s and 1980s. It is likely that the main public health effects of peak oil will be driven by the consequences of an economic downturn. The mechanisms of social and stress-induced illness are now recognized and have been generally accepted. We could therefore reasonably expect a dip in UK life expectancy for the first time since the end of the First World War if such an economic shock were to occur.

There may also, of course, be some beneficial effects from peak oil (Hanlon and McCartney 2008). The availability of individual motorized transport is likely to be lessened, reducing the pressure on climate change after a substantial lag-time. Pollution-driven respiratory illness, road traffic accidents, and the obesity epidemic are all likely to be positively affected by the population increasingly beginning to cycle and walk. There will be an opportunity to move away from the profit-driven, stress-laden globalized system to which we have become accustomed, and this could impact positively on well-being through a range of intermediate factors such as changing work-patterns or increased local community cooperation. Yet there may be negative impacts of such changes, in terms of economic growth, as we explore in the next section.

The modern economy

Concerns about finite resources such as oil are closely linked to the economic model we have adopted because these are interdependent. It is believed that the only way in which our current economic model can be made viable is if it finds the means to continually increase throughput: that is, it must continue to grow, and that growth must be reflected in financial growth. For the current economic system to do well it needs to create extra demand for goods and services, which will themselves have an environmental impact, other things being equal. In order to meet this demand we need a continuous supply of credit, either for consumers or for those who are producing the goods/supplying the services. In order to service the resulting debt there is a need to generate excess returns above the cost of that debt, so we get a spiral of growth built into the economic system. This spiral has to exist to make the current economic model work. Indeed, until the ecological impact of this spiral of growth became evident it was considered to be not just desirable but the main aim of society.

Not to have this growth would cause significant problems in the current context: a no-growth or negative growth model within our current model is not viewed as sustainable by many economists. Lack of growth leads to people being laid off work, which increases calls on the public purse (in terms of unemployment benefit) at exactly the same time as income into the public purse reduces (because fewer taxes are paid). In addition, with inflation and a cap or reduction in public spending, the public sector is plunged into crisis, with salaries reducing in real terms and services suffering because less money is available. All this combines to create a downward spiral that can only be halted and remedied by boosting economic growth – the very thing that may well cease to be possible in future, because of ecological constraints. One such constraint is environmental depletion.

Environmental depletion

Human activity has always accelerated deforestation as land becomes used for arable and pastoral farming. By Roman times Europe was, to all intents and purposes, deforested. This process reached its nadir in the UK in 1750 although the recent planting of trees, largely for commercial purposes, has reversed the process a little. Globally this process of deforestation and loss of mature forest has been accelerated more recently by demand for timber and the clearing of rainforest for commercial crops. From about the mid-1800s, the planet has experienced an unprecedented rate of change in destruction of forests worldwide. Forests in Europe are adversely affected by acid rain and very large areas of Siberia have been harvested since the collapse of the Soviet Union. Since the 1980s, Afghanistan has lost over 70 per cent of its forests. However, it is in the world's great tropical rainforests where the destruction has been most pronounced and where wholesale tree felling is having an adverse effect on biodiversity. Many tropical countries have lost large areas of forest, including almost all of their rainforest. Much of what remains is in the Amazon basin, where the Amazon Rainforest covers more than 600 million hectares. The forests are being destroyed at a pace which mirrors rapid human population growth. Unless significant measures are taken on a worldwide basis to preserve them, by 2030 there will only be ten per cent remaining with another ten per cent in a degraded condition.

Generally, the removal or destruction of significant areas of forest cover has resulted in reduced biodiversity, which has many implications for public health. In many countries, deforestation is shaping climate and geography. Deforestation affects the amount of water in the soil and groundwater and the moisture in the atmosphere. Forests also help to retain topsoil intact and support considerable biodiversity, providing valuable habitat for wildlife. Moreover, forests foster medicinal conservation with forest biotopes being a major, irreplaceable source of new drugs. Deforestation can destroy genetic variations, such as crop resistance, irretrievably. We are also witnessing the loss of fertile soil, with implications for agriculture and food supply. At a planetary level, rich soils are to be found where one finds evidence of glacial or volcanic activity, both of which release essential minerals that are then broken down by weather and taken up by plants. In this sense, Australia and Central West Africa, which have never seen glaciations or volcanic activity, are barren and are being made worse by human activity. For example, over-tillage of soil destroys its structure while over-cropping strips it of tilth and minerals. Globally, over half of the nitrogen and phosphorous which finds its way onto soil is from artificial sources. The planet loses vast quantities of soil every year. For example, during 2010 about 20 billion tonnes of soil found its way into the South China and Yellow Seas because there is not enough forest vegetation to hold the soil in place. Similarly, 70 per cent of all usable fresh water is intercepted, diverted and used for human purposes.

In sum, the environmental and economic challenges outlined above represent major threats to human health. The scale of human activity and the stress that it is causing our home planet is becoming better known. For the first time in the history of our species, human activity is having an impact on the future direction of the biosphere, our survival and that of many other species. From this point of view the impact of the human species on the Earth can be compared to that of an ice age or the impact of a huge asteroid.

Exponential growth = planetary overload

The key point is that our current phase of development has been fuelled by exponential rises in population, energy use and resource consumption. This is not sustainable and the current pattern of growth will have to come to an end, sooner or later. The vital question is whether we can make a transition to a more stable state without going through a major catastrophic collapse, with devastating implications for human health and well-being. What is clear is that the current state of affairs, which depends on exponential growth in the economy and use of vital natural resources, cannot continue indefinitely in the context of a finite planet. The problem is that we humans are not good at recognizing when we are about to reach the peak of a boom phase of growth and move into crash: we do not, in other words, understand the implications of exponential growth. This can be illustrated using the simple thought experiment shown in Box 8.1.

Box 8.1   A thought experiment on exponential growth

Imagine that a bacterium is placed on a nutrient agar plate at nine o'clock in the morning. It reproduces every minute, so at one minute past nine there are two bacteria; at two minutes past, there are four; at three minutes past, eight, and so on. At twelve noon the last division will take place, the plate will be full, all food supplies exhausted, and the whole colony will die. Now, the question is, at what point would a sentient bacterium appreciate that there is an impending crisis?

At 11 a.m., a mere hour away from high noon, the plate would still look empty and no anxiety would be felt. The same would be true at 11.30. Even at 11.55 a.m., five minutes away from the final division that swamps the plate, the surface area remains mostly unoccupied. Only one thirty-second of the surface will have bacterial colonies. Yet such is the power of exponential growth (the ability to grow by multiplying and not just adding) that, by noon minus four minutes, the plate will be one sixteenth covered, while by noon minus three minutes it will be one eighth covered.

By noon minus two minutes the plate will still only be a quarter covered, which means that optimistic bacteria would be able to point to three-quarters of the plate as empty and argue that continuing growth is both possible and desirable. Even at noon minus one minute, the plate is still half empty. Yet sixty seconds later the whole colony dies.

It is now known that the carrying capacity of the Earth to sustain life in the long term was surpassed by human demands sometime in the 1980s (Catton 1982; Butler 2004). This assumes that all of the Earth's capacity is available for human use, which it clearly is not. In recent years it has become more apparent that aspects of the Earth's biodiversity create resilience and stability in various ecosystems. Some argue that it is prudent, since these processes are not well understood, to leave a significant ecological 'buffer' as an insurance policy. Such a buffer is not linear in nature since small proportions of the biosphere contain large proportions of its species. Using the Brundtland Commission's suggestion of a 12 per cent buffer, it appears that humans overran the carrying capacity of the Earth in the early 1970s: by 1999 the extent of the overshoot was 40 per cent. These data say nothing about the rate at which resources are being depleted and so cannot suggest how long remaining biosphere resources will be able to continue in this way.

Economic and environmental collision

The public health community needs to be aware that collision between the economy and the environment now seems inevitable. Economic systems depend on the natural world for resources and for ecological 'services', such as that provided by the climate system but now disrupted by human greenhouse gas emissions (Kickbusch 1989). Any economy that does not respect environmental limits in the long term, therefore, will suffer a backlash that will undermine its ability to operate (with all the attendant social, economic and health costs such a backlash entails). It may be that the backlash will arise only after limits have been breached for some time. How might we respond? A decrease in population would help but will probably not be sought for a number of complex social, economic and cultural reasons. In any case, population decrease will probably occur with a global demographic transition. It may be possible to reduce consumption, especially in already affluent nations. However, modern societies' enduring commitment to economic growth and cultural values of materialism, individualism and consumerism mean that this will probably be difficult and unpopular (Urry 2010). Also, in the current economic model, reduced consumption leads to stagflation and deflation. This suggests that emerging from crisis (economic and ecological) through conventional economics is not plausible (Kovel 2007).

Many people, including the public health community, may turn to technology in the hope that it will help 'square the circle'. However, if we look a little more closely at the scale of the challenge, it becomes clear that technology on its own cannot provide the solution (Jackson 2009).We have a global population of about 7 billion, an average level of affluence of US$8,000 and for every $1,000 of goods and services we consume using current technology, a carbon dioxide emission level of 0.5 tonnes. That equates to annual CO_2 emissions of 28 billon tonnes per year. In order to stabilize CO_2 emissions we need to emit fewer than 5 billion tonnes of CO_2 by 2050 (given a likely population of 9 billion people at this time). This gives a carbon allowance of 0.6 tonnes per person. To put this in context, that is much less than the present carbon footprint per person in India. At today's level of wealth this translates into a carbon footprint of 0.1 tonnes per $1,000 of income: a five-fold improvement in technological efficiency. While this would be difficult it is not beyond our means, if we are focused and devoted to pursuing that goal.

It gets tougher, however, if we factor in economic growth over the world by (say) 2–3 per cent in developed countries and by 5–10 per cent in developing countries, who are seeking to catch up with western standards of consumption (and note that Africa is excluded from this calculation). If we go down that route then we need to get the carbon content of consumption down to less than 0.03 tonnes per $1,000 which represents an elevenfold decrease on current western European average impact (Jackson 2009). If we put a growth figure into the equation to reflect the desire to eradicate poverty (not solely but especially in Africa) the efficiency gains required from technology are higher still. Jackson's (2009) complex but important analysis leads to two logical conclusions. If we are to be able to achieve decarbonization at the same time as having economic growth, the factors of technological improvement required will be huge, not something we have ever been able to achieve before, and have to happen very rapidly over the whole world. Alternatively, we may have to revisit our belief that economic growth is a good thing and/or consider different forms of economic arrangements that would allow human needs to be met within ecological constraints in a viable manner.

Contraction and convergence

It has been calculated that a world of more than nine billion people will require an 80–90 per cent reduction in carbon use by rich countries and drastic reductions in many other forms of consumption, to avoid worsening of existing problems. If sustainability and global equity is to be a goal, we will have to achieve 'contraction' in the richer world and 'convergence' with the poorer world. The phrase 'contraction and convergence' has primarily been used as a response to the threat of runaway climate change (Meyer 2000), and is one with which public health practitioners need to be familiar. Meyer's argument is that the whole world needs a contraction in the production of atmospheric carbon dioxide, which is an output of increased industrialization and economic growth. Rich and poor nations must eventually converge in their carbon production, to avoid nothing less than climate catastrophe. Less developed nations must be allowed to develop – so their carbon use goes up – while industrialized and post industrial nations must make substantial reductions (Meyer 2000). Failure to contract and converge will have health consequences that may be hard to predict but will probably include the loss of agricultural land, severe storms and flooding, forest fires, hunger and forced economic migration, and so on. Contraction and convergence is, of course, another form of redistribution on a global scale, and the concept can apply to other resources and not just the carbon that affluent societies depend on.

Conclusions

This chapter has pointed to the multiple pathways between resource depletion, environmental change, exponential economic growth, and human health and well-being. It thus concludes the part of the book that has drawn together some of the many strands of evidence which indicate that 'modern' society is undergoing profound change. Chapter 4 described how social inequalities in health are increasing, despite decades of research and a considerable number of policy interventions. Chapter 5 explained the (potentially damaging) influence of modern culture and human health and well-being. This enables us to understand problems such as obesity, addictive behaviour and the loss of well-being (described in Chapter 6) as unlike other public health problems for which there are technical solutions. They have developed at the population level because we are apparently biologically and psychologically 'hard wired' in a way that does not entirely suit the modern world in which we live. We are 'stone-agers in the fast lane', to use Nesse's (2005) evocative phrase. Nor have we as yet responded meaningfully to the overarching and interconnected problems of sustainability highlighted by this chapter.

It seems that some of our most intractable health, social and global problems are the product of modernity. These problems have been a long time coming and they have their roots in the deep social, cultural and economic underpinnings of modern society. What are the public health implications of the analysis set out in this part of the book? We might imagine a future where wars are fought so that some countries can maintain current lifestyles (for some of their population). We can probably also imagine greater individualism, verging on selfishness, leading to civil unrest. We can even imagine our civilization collapsing just as others have done before us (Diamond 2005; Homer-Dixon 2006). It goes without saying that these kinds of outcomes should be avoided, as far as possible. A plausible conclusion is that while technological improvement will be essential to mitigate the health and social effects of climate change and other global problems briefly outlined above, there will inevitably be considerable reductions in the level of and change in the nature of consumption. Conventional economic growth will either stop because we create another kind of economic model or it will collapse due to ecological pressures. There are also likely to be significant cultural shifts as to what a 'good life' looks like.

In the society of the future, people will still have material and non-material needs. There will still be economic entities that seek to meet those human needs, but there are also likely to be more community based enterprises that are designed not for profit but to meet specific local needs. The economic viability of entities is unlikely to be predicated on growth, unless their growth displaces other economic activity. Efficiency of production (a quintessentially modern term) will remain important, in that it requires the development of technologies to radically decarbonize and dematerialize production and consumption. Trade will still be present and necessary but is likely to be of a lower volume than is currently the case. Living standards, in terms of the possession of goods, may well fall but this does not automatically mean that well-being in general will decrease. It will be harder to be obese in this changed world, partly because of the price of essentials like food, but also because of a reduction in fossil fuel-sourced mobility.

As noted in the introductory chapter to this book, the human species has experienced profound challenges to its ingenuity in the past and has found creative solutions to overcome them. In the UK and other affluent parts of the world we will all have to 'downshift' to achieve a sustainable way of life – the rich more than the poor – while at the same time re-orientating our individual and collective lives away from the materialism, consumerism and individualism that harm well-being (Hanlon and Carlisle 2010). This is not an invitation to the public health community to indulge in a generalized pessimism about the future, or to advocate some return to a pre-modern way of life (McCartney and Hanlon 2008). On the contrary: we have much to cherish and preserve from the positive aspects of modernity, and much to learn about what really contributes to a good and sustainable quality of life, for the individual and for society. The public health community has a vital role to play in working creatively to imagine and then help bring about an approach to life that enables all of us to 'use less stuff' *and* have better levels of health and well-being (Marks et al. 2006; Simms and Smith 2008). That creative and imaginative work is the focus for the final section of this book. Nevertheless, this is a huge task and one that requires the ingenuity and effort of the entire public health community. We will need to think and act differently. In the concluding chapters we merely begin to scratch the surface of what might be possible.

References

Brown, L.R. (1996) *State of the World 1996: A Worldwatch Institute Report on Progress Toward a Sustainable Society*. New York: W.W. Norton & Company.

Butler, C.D. (2004) Human carrying capacity and human health. *Public Library of Medicine/Public Library of Science*, 1(3): e55.

Catton, W.R. (1982) *Overshoot: The Ecological Basis of Revolutionary Change*. Chicago: University of Illinois Press.

Costello, A., Abbas, M., Allen, A. et al. (2009) Managing the health effects of climate change. *Lancet*, 373: 1693–733.

Davis, S.J., Caldeira, K. and Matthews, H.D. (2010) Future CO_2 emissions and climate change from existing energy infrastructure. *Science*, 329: 1330–3.

Diamond, J. (2005) *How Societies Choose to Fail or Succeed*. London: Pengun.

Haines, A., Kovats, R.S., Campbell-Lendrum, D. and Corvalan, C. (2006) Climate change and human health: impacts, vulnerability, and mitigation. *Lancet*, 367: 2101–9.

Hanlon, P. and Carlisle, S. (2010) Reorienting public health: rhetoric, challenges and possibilities for sustainability. *Critical Public Health*, 20(3): 299–309.

Hanlon, P. and McCartney, G. (2008) Peak oil: will it be public health's greatest challenge? *Public Health*, 122: 647–52.

Homer-Dixon, T. (2000) *The Ingenuity Gap: Facing the Economic, Environmental, and Other Challenges of an Increasingly Complex and Unpredictable World*. London: Jonathan Cape.

Hubbert, M.K. (1945) Energy from fossil fuels. *Science*, 109: 103–9.

Human Development Report (2007/2008) *Fighting Climate Change: Human Solidarity in a Divided World*. New York: United Nations Development Programme.

Intergovernmental Panel on Climate Change (2007) *Fourth Assessment Report*. New York: Cambridge University Press.

Jackson, T. (2009) *Prosperity Without Growth? The Transition to a Sustainable Economy*. London: Sustainable Development Commission.

Kickbusch, I. (1989) Approaches to an ecological base to public health. *Health Promotion International*, 4: 265–8.

Kovel, J. (2007) *The Enemy of Nature: The End of Capitalism or the End of the World?* New York: Zed Books.

Kunstler, J.H. (2005) *The Long Emergency: Surviving the Converging Catastrophes of the Twenty-first Century.* London: Atlantic Books.

Lynas, M. (2008) *Six Degrees: Our Future on a Hotter Planet.* London: Harper Perennial.

McCartney, G. and Hanlon, P. (2008) Climate change and rising energy costs: a threat but also an opportunity for a healthier future? *Public Health*, 122: 653–6.

McMichael, A.J., Powles, J.W., Butler, C.D. and Uauy, R. (2007) Food, livestock production, energy, climate change, and health. *Lancet*, 370: 1253–63.

McMichael, A.J., Woodruff, R.E. and Hales, S. (2006) Climate change and human health: present and future risks. *Lancet*, 367: 859–69.

Mackenbach, J.P. (2007) Global environmental change and human health: a public health research agenda. *Journal of Epidemiology and Community Health*, 61: 92–4.

Marks, N., Abdallah, A., Simms, A. and Thompson, S. (2006) *The (un)Happy Planet Index. An Index of Human Wellbeing and Environmental Impact.* London: nef (new economics foundation).

Meyer, A. (2000) *Contraction and Convergence: The Global Solution to Climate Change.* Totnes: Green Books.

Nesse, R.M. (2005) Natural selection and the elusiveness of happiness. In F.A. Huppert, N. Baylis and B. Keverne (eds) *The Science of Well-being.* Oxford: Oxford University Press.

Roberts, B. (2005) *The End of Oil.* London: Bloomsbury.

Simms, A. and Smith, J. (2008) *Do Good Lives Have to Cost the Earth?* London: Constable & Robinson.

Simms, A., Woodward, D. and Kjell, P. (2004) *Cast Adrift: How the Rich are Leaving the Poor to Sink in a Warming World.* London: new economics foundation (nef).

Smith, J., Schneider, S., Oppenheimer, M. et al. (2009) Assessing dangerous climate change through an update of the Intergovernmental Panel on Climate Change (IPCC): 'reasons for concern'. *Proceedings of the National Academy of Sciences,* 106: 4133–7.

Stern, N. (2007) *The Economics of Climate Change: The Stern Review.* Cambridge: Cambridge University Press.

Stiglitz, J. (2010) *Freefall: America, Free Markets and the Sinking of the World Economy.* Harmondsworth: Allen Lane/Penguin.

United Nations Environment Programme (UNEP) (2009) *Climate Change 2009: Science Compendium.* http://www.unep.org/compendium2009/ (accessed 16 September 2011).

Urry, J. (2010) Consuming the planet to excess. *Theory, Culture and Society*, 27: 191–212.

Wilkinson, P., Smith, K.R., Joffe, M. and Haines, A. (2007) A global perspective on energy: health effects and injustices. *Lancet*, 370: 965–78.

Part 3

The future public health

9 An integrative framework for the future public health

Introduction

Because the future always remains radically open, trying to make detailed predictions is relatively futile. That does not mean, however, that we simply leave everything to fate. There are intentional ways to move forward which will help shape the future. Previous chapters of this book have drawn together some of the many strands of evidence which support the contention that modern society is undergoing a 'change of age' (Hanlon and Carlisle 2008). We have illustrated for example, that obesity, unlike public health problems for which there is a technical solution, has developed at the population level because we are biologically 'hard-wired' in a way that does not suit the modern world of convenient and affordable high calorie food and drinks. The same might be said of our psychological 'wiring' and our loss of well-being (Lane 2000). Humans evolved in closely-knit kinship groups which probably possessed a powerful collective sense of identity, so we now find ourselves ill equipped for the strongly individualized social world created by modernity. In short, many of our most intractable health problems are the product of modernity, which means that the tools of modernity are ill suited to finding solutions.

Looking beyond public health, much of the modern world is confronted with an ingenuity gap – the gulf between a spectrum of problems we encounter and our capacity to devise effective solutions (Homer-Dixon 2000). One pertinent example is the regeneration of disadvantaged inner city areas that have undergone deindustrialization and decline. Such neighbourhoods typically suffer from high unemployment, low levels of amenities or services, high levels of crime, low levels of trust, poor educational outcomes, and much else, including poorer health outcomes. Various governments have, for several decades, attempted area-based regeneration: rebuilding houses then rebuilding them again. Yet the problems apparently remain intractable. Part of the difficulty is that, true to our modern mindset, we approach regeneration as if it were only a material problem. This is not to deny that lack of material resources plays a large role in the problems encountered by people living in such areas. The point is that the material dimension of life inevitably interacts with emotional, aesthetic, moral and spiritual dimensions. For regeneration to be effective, these dimensions also have to be considered, but rarely are. People working in large bureaucratic organizations find it difficult to engage with this wide range of issues because those organizations are not structured to support such an integrated approach. The result is that they continue to spend millions of pounds on housing and the physical environment and are unable to understand why there are only small scale improvements in the health and well-being of populations so targeted. In these settings, it is becoming clearer that what we know how to do is not what needs to be done.

Nevertheless, there is little evidence that our failure to solve the deeper problems created by modernity is causing us to radically change tack. For example, the obesity epidemic is not automatically self-limiting. If left unchecked, it may bring other unforeseeable changes and difficulties. If it is to be reversed without harm, we will probably have to change our whole food economy, the balance of what we eat, and how active we are. This is only likely to happen if we change the way we organize our lives and our society. There is precious little evidence that we are even attempting such change. We are, for example, adapting to and normalizing a much larger body shape. For some, this may be a positive and anti-discriminatory development. For the public health community, it remains problematic because of the implications of unhealthy weight gain for health outcomes and quality of life over the longer term. Equally, for all the rhetoric about abolishing child poverty and addressing social justice, almost all indicators of inequality in the UK are moving in the wrong direction.

We could, on the basis of the four previous waves of public health set out in the first part of this book, be tempted to assume that a fifth wave will develop in a similar way. An alternative view is that the nature of the challenges facing public health at the beginning of the twenty-first century are such that a fifth wave of public health will not appear from its accumulated traditions but rather will emerge from radically different ways of thinking, being and doing. There is evidence that the whole wave of modernity is peaking and is moving into decline. So, to create a fifth wave – the future public health – a dynamic is needed that transcends modernity, while retaining its still valuable aspects. Public health may require a new and more appropriate paradigm with which to navigate the turbulent present and (as yet) unknowable future. Much of this chapter describes some of the possible ingredients of a new paradigm, in the form of key features and a conceptual framework which could be used to underpin the future public health.

Reasons for (cautious) optimism

It is as well to begin this journey into the future with a positive message. With the benefit of hindsight we can identify a number of changes of age over the course of human history, each with a distinctive outer world (social structure, economy, ecology and culture) and inner world (belief system, values, motivations and consciousness) (Rifkin 2009). Resource and population pressures catalysed each change of age (Harrison 1993). To cope, our ancestors developed new outer and inner worlds and the modern age has followed this pattern. So the lesson of history is that human beings have negotiated several changes of age in the past. Can modern society do the same? The ability of modern people to understand, predict and control the natural world has brought undoubted benefits, such as better health, health care, and material prosperity. The challenge that faces us is the need to preserve these benefits while addressing the adverse effects of modernity. However, as noted above, there is little evidence that many people are responding positively, by embracing new forms of thinking or practice. Rather, what can be observed is denial, resistance and passive forms of adaptation, which prop up the existing system (Ereaut and Segnit 2006; Segnit and Ereaut 2007).

Chapter 8 highlighted the danger of societal collapse precipitated by ecological and economic forces inherent in our current trajectory (in particular climate change – Stern 2006; IPCC 2007; Jackson 2009) and peak oil (Roberts 2005). We know, from what happened after the collapse of the Soviet bloc, that this would be a public health disaster. Yet profound societal change is inevitable: this can be made voluntarily to avoid collapse, or involuntarily in response to collapse. Paradoxically, the inevitability of change is a reason for optimism: in such circumstances public health has an opportunity to use the dynamic created by change to bridge some of its most profound ingenuity gaps (Homer-Dixon 2000). The important question, therefore, for anyone who is concerned about the health and well-being of populations is how to support transformational change while sustaining what is necessary from the existing system to ensure the long-term viability of human societies, and other species. A key issue for the public health community in these circumstances is to find a way to think and act effectively in potentially overwhelming circumstances.

Propositions for the future public health

If transformational change that addresses the challenges of sustainability, equity and health is to be achieved then, for all the arguments rehearsed throughout this book, a new and integrative approach will be needed (Hanlon et al. 2010). The future public health will plausibly need to be radically different from today's orthodoxy, while retaining all that is worthwhile in current practice. What will be the plausible features of the future public health if it is to realize this ambition? For now, five key features are suggested:

1   To succeed, the future public health should seek to be **integrative**. That is, public health will play its part in re-integrating dimensions of life that have been effectively separated by modernity itself – the interior and the exterior; the objective and the subjective; the individual and the collective; the good, the true and the beautiful, or science, ethics and aesthetics.

2   The future public health should aspire to be **ecological**. It may take time for a consensus understanding of 'ecological public health' to be agreed and a worthwhile public health practice to emerge but at this stage in its development two dimensions seem to be important. First, a systems perspective is needed to gain insights from the many natural and man-made complex adaptive systems that influence human health and well-being. Second, to the already well established focus on ecosystems in nature, there is a need to expand our awareness of cultural, social and human ecologies.

3   The future public health needs to be **ethical** at two levels. Individual human rights are fundamental but these should be integrated with collective imperatives; in particular, the need for equity and sustainability.

4   To overcome the ingenuity gap, the future public health will require **creativity**. The human imagination, the ability to envision something better, will be a key resource. However, the capacity for creativity seems to be a product of human consciousness and, if public health remains trapped in the consciousness that helped to create our current problems, creativity will be blocked. This suggests that our personal practice and our institutional structures should be consciously designed to unblock the forces that impede creativity.

5   The future public health also needs to be **beautiful** in the sense that it 'raises our spirits' and 'fires our imagination'. Activities and relationships that are beautiful in this sense will have the power to attract others, and will help to maintain the enthusiasm and continuing commitment of those involved.

These positive features are, we hope, likely to constitute the future of our discipline. However, the next section looks to the past in an attempt to describe what might be called the root cause of some of modernity's problems. Any response to our current predicament must be judged in terms of its ability to grapple with the root causes of that predicament, and not just its symptoms. So it may be helpful to think about the nature of modernity and its origins.

Root causes of modernity's problems

Consider the time in history when Galileo joined a small group of those who argued that the earth moved round the sun and not the other way round. In the world of medieval Christianity it was not possible to examine the objective scientific truth of planetary movements without simultaneously challenging ideas of morality (Man and his world as the centrepiece of God's creation, with moral responsibilities [whereas women were responsible for the fall from divine grace]) and beauty (the harmony of the geo-centric universe). Galileo was met by opposition primarily because those who objected had never differentiated what is 'true' (science) from what is 'good' (ethics and morality) and what is 'beautiful' (aesthetics and art).

Part of what made the modern world possible was the ability to examine evidence in order to establish 'truth', without this process threatening morality and aesthetics (the good and the beautiful). In the centuries that followed Galileo, science and its associated technologies brought us multiple benefits. The modern differentiation of the spheres of art, ethics and science set each free to pursue its own path and values. However, this differentiation also allowed an imperialistic form of science to develop and dominate the other spheres by claiming that it alone had access to 'reality', through the objectivity and value-neutrality of the scientific method (an ideology best described as scientism).

Re-integrating the true, the good and the beautiful

The three categories introduced above – the true, the good and the beautiful (or science, ethics and aesthetics) (see Figure 9.1) – are ancient and derive from Platonic thinking (O'Hear 2007). They also resonate with Wilber's (2001)

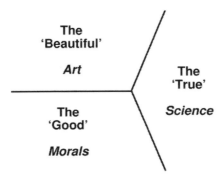

Figure 9.1 Plato and the Good, the True, and the Beautiful.

	Subjective-Interior	Objective-Exterior
Individual level	**I** The inner world	**It** The body, the physical world
Collective level	**We** Culture	**Its** Society

Figure 9.2 Wilber's integral model.

integral model of the four key dimensions of human experience (see Figure 9.2), introduced in Chapters 5 and 6. Such thinking remains relatively unknown within public health, yet provides insights that we need and can put to use.

The idea of the 'true' (i.e. science) corresponds to the right hand column of Wilber's four quadrant model, which deals with the objective, exterior dimensions of life, at both individual and collective levels ('it' and 'its'). Ideas of the 'good' (ethics, morality) and the 'beautiful' (aesthetics, art, creativity) correspond with the left hand column, which deals with the subjective, interior dimensions, at both individual and collective levels ('I' and 'we'). The key point here is that, in everyday life, we tend not to differentiate these dimensions of experience: rather we integrate them naturally, as a matter of course. As an example, imagine that you are an experienced public health worker with a young family, who has been given the opportunity to work for a charity in sub-Saharan Africa. Before accepting you and your family would try to ensure all aspects of the job, arrangements for accommodation, schooling for your children, their safety and health, a possible role for your partner and much else, are properly investigated. In short, you would objectively assess what is 'true' about the proposed venture.

At the same time, you would be likely to ask yourself questions like 'is this the right priority for us at this time?'; 'are there other more important experiences the children need, or would it be good for them to experience another culture and language?', and so on. Again, it is part of human nature to be alert to these issues: what is the 'good' and right thing to do? You and your family would also be sensitive to the aesthetic and creative dimensions of such plans. You would probably ask yourselves whether this would be a 'beautiful' experience, in the sense of giving all of you a chance to live more creatively and expand your awareness. However, considerations of the 'good' and 'beautiful' rarely occur to us in our daily working lives within the dominant systems of modernist institutions. These have yielded a great deal over the years in terms of health and social improvements but the narrowness of their cultural values can douse the commitment and energy of those who join them in order to work for 'the good'. This is why the future public health needs to integrate the true, the good and the beautiful (see Figure 9.3).

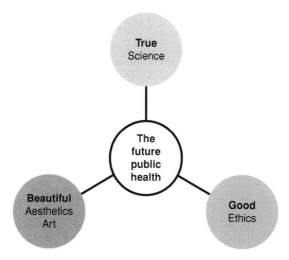

Figure 9.3   The future public health.

The question is, how is this to be accomplished? Public health will need more than current forms of science, ethics and aesthetics. We will also need 'emergent' forms of these (explained below). It is important to emphasize that this approach to public health would still adhere to the rules of evidence-based practice and good science, with no compromise over scientific integrity. It does imply that, in addition to the value we place on the currency of conventional science, other currencies will also be valued. As argued above, these will include systems and ecological insights, qualitative methods and the wisdom that can come from narratives, dialogue, personal experience and pattern recognition. The six dimensional framework (see Figure 9.4) incorporates the components of the future public health that will need to be integrated. A description of these components follows.

1   Current public health science

An examination of the curricula for public health training in the UK suggests that the five basic sciences of public health are epidemiology, biostatistics, environmental science, management science and behavioural/social sciences. Other fields of knowledge include demography, social policy and health economics. Communicable disease control and environmental health together constitute a significant body of knowledge within public health, while skills like health needs assessment, health impact assessments and health equity audits have become increasingly important. Finally, public health needs the skills to critically appraise and evaluate practice and to formulate new

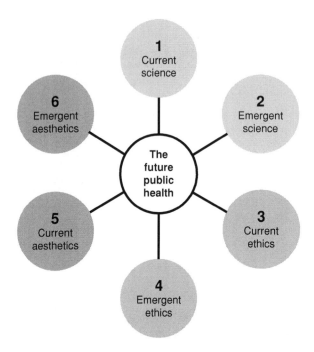

Figure 9.4 Six integrated components.

research. This is a daunting and demanding list. Public health practitioners may feel overwhelmed by their current workload, so our practice stands in need of a greater sense of balance – of the ability to stand back and take a wider view of the landscape wherein we operate, to understand the whole and not just work on the parts.

The problem here is current public health sciences are overly reliant on reductionist approaches in seeking to grapple with the escalating health problems of modernity or emerging ecological threats to health. Reductionism has helped us to understand a great deal about the natural world. It does so by separating out strands of information from reality, which is highly complex, and reducing them to the interactions of their parts. There are numerous ways in which reductionism has proved to be an effective tool for creating understanding which, in turn, has led to interventions that improve our lives. Yet it has limitations: a complex system is always more than the sum of its parts and cannot be explained by reducing it to individual constituents; and the real world has an intra-personal dimension which is missing from the strictly objective world view. Different types of thinking are therefore needed to help explain reality and to help us understand the nature of the health challenges that we face.

2 Emergent sciences for the future public health

Reductionist viewpoints and holistic viewpoints can be thought of as two ends of a spectrum, where each has validity in seeking to describe and explain that complex and multidimensional entity that we (usually) refer to simply as 'reality'. The second component of our future public health framework will use insights and perspectives drawn from the more holistic end of this spectrum. What is 'emergent' is the idea that a much wider range of paradigms, methods and mindsets will inform our science as we confront the problems of a change in age. Consider the example of environmental health, which has long been a pillar of public health and is already beginning to move in a more holistic direction. Its key task has been to determine, assess and measure environmental threats to health which can then be removed; where this proves impossible, populations can be protected by containment or protection. This approach is typically rigorous and reductionist, and none the worse for it.

More recently, awareness of the threat of global ecological hazards to human health has seen the emergence of 'ecological' forms of public health. A number of different approaches to this topic can be discerned within our discipline (Hanlon and Carlisle 2010). Some, for example, have applied a very traditional scientific model to particular issues that will arise from a given rise in global temperature (Haines et al. 2006; Costello et al. 2009). A second approach applies existing public health models of the determinants of heath and modifies them to the new challenges (Nurse et al. 2010). This too has value but tends to suggest that the current repertoire of sciences will be sufficient for the task. A third approach, which adopts a more holistic methodology, is beginning to emerge, focused on whole systems (natural and man-made) that interact with each other to affect human health (Kickbusch 1998; Rayner 2009). All three approaches have merit and the skilled public health practitioner of the future will need to discern which is required in what circumstance. We will need to learn to integrate reductionist and holistic perspectives with other scientific insights that have yet to fully emerge, such as chaos and complexity theories and recent developments in the cognitive sciences. We will need open minds and the capacity to adapt to the (formerly) unconventional (Leischow and Milstein 2006).

3 Current ethics

The roots of medical ethics may be traced to physicians in antiquity (Hippocrates), and early Islamic and Christian teachings. During the Enlightenment, medical ethics emerged as a more self-conscious discourse becoming formalized, in the period since the Second World War, into codes of ethics under the umbrella of statements about human rights. Public health ethics has its roots in the four foundational principles of medical ethics (i.e. autonomy; beneficence; non-maleficence; justice) but has also attempted to create a distinctive set of principles that apply to population health interventions rather than individually applied treatments (see, for example, the 2007 Nuffield Council Report on Bioethics). While helpful, current ethics fail to address some of the truly difficult ethical questions with which the future public health will have to grapple.

4 Emergent ethics

The great achievement of current ethics, built on a long tradition, is that it encourages us to place a high value on each human life and has invested each person (irrespective of status or circumstance) with fundamental human rights. So, when we speak of an emergent ethics it is vital that this does not weaken or dilute the achievements of current ethics. Nevertheless, current ethics in public health does not adequately address the two major and linked issues of social justice and ecological public health.

Consider, for example, the challenge of 'contraction and convergence' (Meyer 2000). This is a concept that has been developed in response to global warming and other environmental threats. The idea is simple. The world needs a contraction in output of carbon dioxide but for all to buy into such an agreement it must be transparently just: hence the need for convergence. Less developed nations must be allowed to develop, which may mean increased carbon utilization, while industrialized and post industrial nations must make substantial reductions. However, an ethical framework which ensures global justice and equity while safeguarding the rights of individuals has yet to emerge. This will be a key challenge if the world is not to face runaway climate change and collapse.

Our track record on global justice is variable. For example, there have been campaigns and international agreements to cancel debt and reduce the flow of money from the world's poor to the world's rich. Yet in 2006 nearly $500 billion more was transferred from poor to rich countries, than flowed the other way (Simms et al. 2006). This is an ethical and moral issue and should be addressed for those reasons. However, because of the dominance of scientism and economism, moral and ethical arguments often hold little sway. Current public health ethics have almost nothing to say about how such examples of social injustice are to be addressed.

The challenge of reducing inequalities needs to be linked to the ethical challenges of over consumption and sustainability. The rich have been successful in resisting appeals for greater equity but the point about problems like climate change is that we will all be affected and we all need to participate if a solution is to be found. Unless a new form of ethics emerges that sees the connected nature of all people (indeed, of all life), we will find it hard to achieve transformational change in inequalities. A move in the direction described above implies a change in values and mindset. Our understanding of who we are as people and those to whom we relate with care and inclusion has changed in the past and will change again (Rifkin 2009). The challenges are great, but so is our individual and collective capacity to respond: we have perhaps never been so close to the development of an empathic civilization as we now are. However, changing human consciousness takes us into the territory of the final two components of the future public health framework.

5   Current aesthetics

This part of the framework is probably the most unfamiliar to public health. We talk about combining the science and art of public health but seldom define the latter. Since *Homo sapiens* emerged we have been engaged in creating: making tools; painting the walls of caves; crafting personal decorations; and much more, possibly as part of the human impulse to create meaning. Without creativity our work can become commonplace and without meaning. Yet in modern culture even this aspect of our humanity has been commandeered for instrumental purposes and commodified within the consumer marketplace. So, art becomes of value if it is part of regeneration or therapy but not for its own sake or for its capacity to inspire or be meaningful.

6   Emergent aesthetics

The scale of the challenges facing human health and well-being is clear. The need for transformational change to meet these challenges is equally clear. As human beings we will need to create new art, stories, myths, symbols and much else to help us make the inner and outer transformations that will be needed. We use the term 'emergent' because, while we are sure change is coming, the manner in which we will respond in our individual and collective imaginations will need to emerge from a continuing and dynamic process of discovery and creativity. So, activities in this dimension of the framework will centre on being fully human: being creative; being playful; developing consciousness; fostering empathy, and much else. Creativity is important because it is part of our nature and, as positive psychology has shown, we are often at our happiest and most fulfilled when lost in the flow and challenge of creativity (Csikszentmihalyi 1990). It is also from our creative selves that solutions to our most profound problems often arise. Creativity is also important because it balances some of the more intellectual and instrumental modes of being that tend to dominate our working lives.

Conclusion: an integrative framework for health

The nature of the problems confronting public health call for a different approach to integration than our current ability to combine core public health sciences with insights from the behavioural and social sciences. The focus of this chapter has been on a wider and deeper approach to integration, given that – as we explained above – separation, differentiation and fragmentation appear fundamental to the mindset that has created those problems. So we end this chapter with a tentative summary of the elements that need to be integrated as we work towards the future public health. The integrative framework for health shown in Figure 9.5 suggests that the future public health will be part of an emerging way of life that requires different ways of thinking, being and doing. The framework is descriptive, but it also moves towards prescription. Current public health science will need to be integrated with

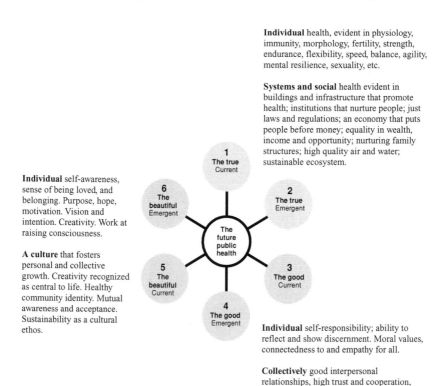

Individual health, evident in physiology, immunity, morphology, fertility, strength, endurance, flexibility, speed, balance, agility, mental resilience, sexuality, etc.

Systems and social health evident in buildings and infrastructure that promote health; institutions that nurture people; just laws and regulations; an economy that puts people before money; equality in wealth, income and opportunity; nurturing family structures; high quality air and water; sustainable ecosystem.

Individual self-awareness, sense of being loved, and belonging. Purpose, hope, motivation. Vision and intention. Creativity. Work at raising consciousness.

A culture that fosters personal and collective growth. Creativity recognized as central to life. Healthy community identity. Mutual awareness and acceptance. Sustainability as a cultural ethos.

1 The true Current

6 The beautiful Emergent

2 The true Emergent

The future public health

5 The beautiful Current

3 The good Current

4 The good Emergent

Individual self-responsibility; ability to reflect and show discernment. Moral values, connectedness to and empathy for all.

Collectively good interpersonal relationships, high trust and cooperation, mutual awareness and acceptance, social justice, strong ethical principles. Ethics arises from empathic concern. Intergenerational justice and empathy.

Figure 9.5 An integrative framework for health.

emergent science to inform future thinking and practice around individual and social health, and the various natural and social systems that support these. Our ethical thinking and practice will need to integrate individual rights and responsibilities with collective rights and responsibilities. We will need a greater awareness of the vital role of aesthetics in our individual lives and the culture in which we live. But the point is that none of these desirable changes can stand alone: for example, our thinking and practice with regard to the issue of sustainability will need to integrate insights from the domains of science, ethics and aesthetics. If we continue to separate and differentiate these, granting worth to one while devaluing the others, we are unlikely to succeed in navigating the many changes facing our society.

So progress needs to be made in all six segments simultaneously and not just in one. However, the framework does not imply that 'health' equals success in all areas: that would be utopian. Equally, the framework is not suggesting that those with major problems (including disease and/or disability) cannot be healthy. Rather, the integrative framework is a summary of activities that will need to come together to create the type of concept of health and well-being required for the future. This integrative approach may seem radical but we are confident that it will, over time, and for all the reasons set out in earlier chapters of this book, become the new 'second nature' for public health practitioners. In the next chapter we explore the question of how this might happen, as we apply the integrative framework to some major public health challenges, and to a future NHS.

References

Costello, A., Abbas, M., Allen, A. et al. (2009) Managing the health effects of climate change. *Lancet*, 373: 1693–733.

Csikszentmihalyi, M. (1990) *Flow: The Psychology of Optimal Experience*. New York: Harper and Row.

Ereaut, G. and Segnit, N. (2006) *Warm Words: How are we Telling the Climate Story and Can we Tell it Better?* London: Institute for Public Policy Research.

Haines, A., Kovats, R.S., Campbell-Lendrum, D. and Corvalan, C. (2006) Climate change and human health: impacts, vulnerability, and mitigation. *Lancet*, 367: 2101–9.

Hanlon, P. and Carlisle, S. (2008) Do we face a third revolution in human history? If so, how will Public Health respond? *Journal of Public Health*, 30(4): 355–61.

Hanlon, P. and Carlisle, S. (2010) Re-orienting public health: rhetoric, challenges and possibilities for sustainability. *Critical Public Health*, 20(3): 299–309.

Hanlon, P., Carlisle, S., Reilly, D., Lyon, A. and Hannah, M. (2010) Enabling well-being in a time of radical change: integrative public health for the 21st century. *Public Health*, 124: 305–12.

Harrison, P. (1993) *The Third Revolution: Population, Environment and a Sustainable World*. London: Penguin Books.

Homer-Dixon, T. (2000) *The Ingenuity Gap: Facing the Economic, Environmental, and Other Challenges of an Increasingly Complex and Unpredictable Future*. New York: Vintage Books.

IPCC (Intergovernmental Panel on Climate Change) (2007) *Fourth Assessment Report*. New York: Cambridge University Press.

Jackson, T. (2009) *Prosperity Without Growth? The Transition to a Sustainable Economy*. London: Sustainable Development Commission.

Kickbusch, I. (1989) Approaches to an ecological base to public health. *Health Promotion International*, 4: 265–8.

Lane, R.E. (2000) *The Loss of Happiness in Market Democracies*. London: Yale University Press.

Leischow, S.J. and Milstein, B. (2006) Systems thinking and modeling for public health practice. *American Journal of Public Health*, 96(3): 403–5.

Meyer, A. (2000) *Contraction and Convergence: The Global Solution to Climate Change*. Totnes: Green Books.

Nuffield Council on Bioethics (2007) *Public Health: Ethical Issues*. London: Nuffield Council on Bioethics.

Nurse, J., Basher, D., Bone, A. and Bird, W. (2010) An ecological approach to promoting population mental health and well-being – a response to the challenge of climate change. *Perspectives in Public Health*, 130(1): 27–33.

O'Hear, A. (ed.) (2007) *Philosophy: The Good, The True and The Beautiful* (Special Supplement 47). London: Royal Institute of Philosophy.

Rayner, G. (2009) Conventional and ecological public health. *Public Health*, 123: 587–91.

Rifkin, J. (2009) *The Empathic Civilization: The Race to Global Consciousness in a World in Crisis*. Cambridge: Polity Press.

Roberts, B. (2005) *The End of Oil*. London: Bloomsbury.

Segnit, N. and Ereaut, G. (2007) *Warm Words II: How the Climate Story is Evolving and the Lessons we Can Learn for Encouraging Public Action*. London: Energy Saving Trust and Institute for Public Policy Research.

Simms, A., Moran, D. and Chowler, P. (2006) *The UK Interdependence Report: How the World Sustains the Nation's Lifestyles and the Price it Pays*. London: new economics foundation (nef).

Stern, N. (2006) *The Economics of Climate Change: The Stern Review*. Cambridge: Cambridge University Press.

Wilber, K. (2001) *A Theory of Everything: An Integral Vision for Business, Politics, Science and Spirituality*. Dublin: Gateway.

10 Applying the integrative framework to the major public health challenges and the future NHS

Introduction

In earlier chapters, a series of escalating public health challenges were explored including widening inequalities, obesity (Foresight Report 2007), addiction-related harm (Alexander 2008), and loss of well-being (Lane 2000; James 2008). These, together with the health threats of ecological collapse, are referred to in the sections below as the major public health challenges. For each of these major challenges the argument has been made that conventional public health approaches fail because they fail to recognize that the problems are manifestations of modernity itself. In response, Chapter 9 proposed a series of key features that will help shape the future public health. Thus, the future public health was envisioned as **integrative** as it brings together all six elements of the model: integrating the good, the true and the beautiful. It was envisioned as **ecological** in its awareness of ecological limits to growth and the need to engage with but not pretend to understand and control complex systems. The future public health will understand that the manner in which the modern era has exploited energy has direct links to, for example, our use of the car and our food systems. A change in the ecology of energy use is our best opportunity to reverse the obesity epidemic. The **beauty** of a possible future that has greater health, equity and sustainability is part of what will raise our spirits and fire our imagination. The need for a vision is an important part of achieving positive change. The approach is **ethical** at two levels. It respects individual human rights and is not coercive. Nonetheless, it anticipates a change in human consciousness that is global in its concern and future oriented. The future public health will also require **creativity**, as this highlights the need for personal practice and institutional structures that foster creativity.

The above elements of the future public health apply to the *discipline* of public health, so to this list must be added a further two features that relate more specifically to the future public health *practitioner*. The future public health will need to be **embodied** in the sense that it will require practitioners to be the change that they want to see in the world. Consequently, it will also need to be **reflexive**. That is, practitioners will become increasingly self-aware (aware of their own mindset and worldview), open to the need for new learning and the ability to understand other perspectives, and able to change their own practice in response. Chapter 11 focuses more closely on the future public health practitioner.

In this chapter we use the integrative framework to consider what integrative and ecological responses to the major public health challenges might look like. We then apply this integrative and ecological model to health care, in a future NHS.

Applying the integrative and ecological framework to major public health challenges

1 Current science

Work conducted by the various sciences that underpin public health practice will continue to have relevance. More will be discovered about each of the major public health challenges and this will add to the evidence base for

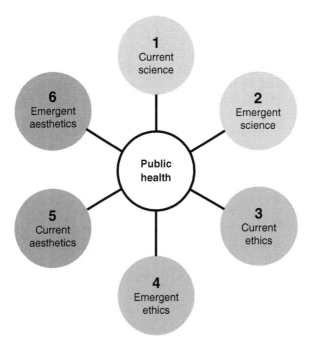

Figure 10.1 Applying the integrative and ecological framework to the major public health challenges.

action. However, unless these insights are integrated with other dimensions of the framework, the ingenuity gap will persist: insights from conventional sciences face diminishing returns in terms of what they are able to add to existing knowledge, using purely scientific methods of enquiry (Jones 2000).

2 Emergent science

Systems-based analysis has already established the links between obesity and the increasing use of oil for transport and food production (Roberts 2005; Foresight Report 2007). It is probable that the only force powerful enough to reverse the obesity epidemic will be the emergence of a society that moves beyond current energy intensive approaches to agriculture and food production and makes the car a less central part of life. Addressing the challenge of peak oil and the need to decarbonize the global economy (or use carbon in a different way) provide the only realistic way in which this might be achieved. In turn, these changes require a move away from economic growth as the central aim of most societies. Such a change in emphasis would take the wind out of the sails of consumerism, thus allowing people to slow their pace on the 'hedonic treadmill', pursuing short-term gratification at the expense of long-term well-being. That treadmill also needs to become less valued, which would encourage people to jump off and pursue more worthwhile alternatives. There would be less money in circulation and carbon would have to be shared equitably to ensure that limits were observed.

The result could be a reduction in inequalities in income which may have beneficial impacts on inequalities in health (although greed in some sectors of society may well be profoundly resistant and possibly ineradicable). The pace of life could become slower but people could well feel less isolated and pressured. Finally, the economic system may shift its focus, so that it becomes more economical to grow food locally and to manufacture goods closer to the point of consumption (thus reducing energy costs for transport). Such changes could provide meaningful work for many who, in recent decades, have been excluded. Recognizing the links between energy, food, transport, economic growth, obesity, well-being and inequalities allows us to imagine a radically different set of interactions which could become the emergent qualities of the change of age. An array of far less desirable futures is of course possible, but this fact does not reduce our responsibility to use these insights to work for a healthier, more equitable and sustainable future. The interdependencies between problems could lead either to spirals of rapid decline, or to positive transformation.

3 Current ethics

The liberal market economy dictates that almost all goods and increasing proportions of services are seen as commodities; in this context, it is assumed that the ethics of the market place dictate what is produced, promoted, sold and consumed. Some have attempted to bring a social justice perspective to bear on this argument and have argued for fair trade policies and practice. Others have suggested that regulation and taxation should be used as instruments of policy to promote greater equity and less waste. However, these still tend to be minority voices: the ethics of the market place are still dominant. It seems that our concept of justice remains focused primarily on individual freedoms, and the promise that continued economic growth provides the 'rising tide' that 'lifts all boats'. Yet there are now grave doubts that the current economic model is sustainable; evidence suggests not. Those guided by ethical concerns for others will want to minimize the enormous potential for harm that will accompany any collapse of our current way of living.

4 Emergent ethics

This dimension of the framework could lead to the conclusion that healthy, equitable and sustainable ways of living should be both an individual and communal goal. This means that our use of energy and consumables has to decrease overall while becoming more equitably distributed. It seems plausible that only a transparently just, global agreement on such matters will be acceptable worldwide. This suggests that a collective debate is needed as to what constitutes a good life in a good society. That life and that society could be rich in many aspects (time, relationships and creative work) even if it has less in the way of disposable material goods. We need to remember that possible futures already exist, the future will be created through human activity and its making will change both our destination and ourselves. The value base we bring to bear on the coming transition is therefore vitally important: either we are genuinely all in this together, or we are not.

5 Current aesthetics

The manner in which the world might change so that it is more successful in raising our spirits and firing our imagination can be illustrated by focusing on one key 'commodity' in modern life: food. The point is that food is never simply a commodity. As explained in Chapter 5, the production and consumption of food is intrinsically rich in meaning in all human societies: it is used for ritual purposes, for celebration, for social interaction, to promote family solidarity, to demonstrate care for others, and much more. The preparation of food and its presentation has long been an expression of human creativity, although this has been suppressed to a large extent by the industrialized processes around food production found in modern society. The 'Slow Food Movement' recognizes this aesthetic and meaningful dimension of food and seeks to promote a more mindful engagement with its preparation and consumption. It seems clear that an appreciation of the aesthetic dimension of food is integral to its healthy and sustainable use. If this is the case for food, it is plausible for other forms of consumption and all aspects of work. A slower, more creative and mindful approach could transform our sense of well-being and enhance our sense of connection to others.

6 Emergent aesthetics

This dimension of the framework reminds us that our engagement with others actually helps us to become more aware of ourselves, in relation to each other and the planet. Many people in modern society are already aware of this, and public health needs to join their number. We should also be aware that this new aesthetic must emerge in the presence of the old one, so its path is not assured. Modernity is implicated in the creation of the major public health challenges, in that they are a fundamental manifestation of our inner life (our mindset and worldview) and our outer life (the structure of our society and culture). Therefore the tools of modernity (government programmes, public health interventions, social marketing or whatever) are unlikely to make a fundamental difference.

In short, the major public health challenges provide us with both threat and opportunity. The opportunity is that the waning of materialism, individualism, consumerism, scientism and economism could help a different form of society to emerge, one in which the major public health challenges listed above have been reversed. The vision to work towards is a world with a stable population, sustainable forms of production and consumption, lower levels of depression and anxiety, less obesity, higher levels of well-being, more human association and humane organizations, less addiction and greater equity. Those who think this inconceivable might reflect on just how 'imaginable' a (relatively) clean and modern city of the twenty-first century, with all its facilities, would have been to a nineteenth century agricultural worker, forced off the land to work in the early factories of the industrial revolution. The integrative framework provides a starting point for public health to play its part in grasping the opportunities inherent in the transitions we face.

Applying an integrative and ecological framework to the future NHS

To clarify the framework introduced in Chapter 9 and illustrated in Figure 10.1 above, its implications for the NHS are addressed below, as an example of how it might influence practice. By working through this example, different solutions to the current approaches to the economic downturn and financial pressures on the UK health service become possible. Currently

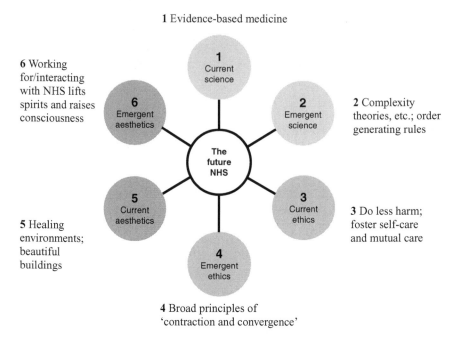

1 Evidence-based medicine

6 Working for/interacting with NHS lifts spirits and raises consciousness

2 Complexity theories, etc.; order generating rules

5 Healing environments; beautiful buildings

3 Do less harm; foster self-care and mutual care

4 Broad principles of 'contraction and convergence'

Figure 10.2 Applying the integrative and ecological framework to the NHS.

we use either financially-led salami-slicing of budgets or rationalistically in-spired ideas about efficiency in order to get more out for the same or less input. We offer here a different perspective: one based on more ecological and in-tegrated forms of thinking and practice which could provide a stimulus for fresh dialogue on contemporary challenges. What would the NHS look like if it adopted more ecological and integrated forms of thinking and practice across the currently fragmented domains of the true (science), the good (ethics) and the beautiful (aesthetics)? The six dimensions of the framework shown in Figure 10.2 are explored in turn. We then consider how close the NHS is to adopting such a model, and whether any other organizations 'do it better'.

1 Current science

Reductionism as currently practised in health care has produced many posi-tives, such as the development of randomized control trials; rigorous proto-cols; evidence-based clinical guidelines; and so on. However, it has failed to fully address the unintended harms caused by health care, the loss of much patient autonomy, the challenge of multiple pathologies, and the challenge of eventual physical decline and inevitable death. It has also arguably lost sight of what might be called the 'art of care' and in the process neglected some of the broader human needs of both patients and professional practitioners.

2 Emergent and ecological science

Other forms of scientific thinking (systems theories, complexity theories, insights from the social sciences) are also of value in helping us explain reality. Complexity theory and chaos theory study systems whose complexity defies accurate predictions of their future, but which nevertheless exhibit underlying patterns (Gleick 1987). Understanding underlying patterns can help us cope in an increasingly complex world. Insights from systems, chaos and complexity theories, when combined with insights from the social sciences, would enable us to understand the NHS as a complex, adaptive system that operates in a shifting cultural environment. In consequence, greater attention would be directed to the 'order generating rules' that create structure and dictate functions. System science insights would also be combined with socio-cultural insights to allow the system to become self aware, learn and develop (Capra 1997). Systems thinking is now becoming commonplace in some parts of the NHS; the problem is that the system is still perceived as an objective reality, and not the subjective construction of all its participants.

3 Current ethics

Two of the foundational principles of conventional ethics need to be addressed. First, the injunction to: 'do no harm'. Iatrogenic disease is far too common in the UK health service and the more treatments that are administered the greater the harm that may result. The new NHS will need a deeper dialogue between patients and professionals about the desirability of ensuring that, in particular contexts, less rather than more is done – fewer procedures and less treatment in some cases. The current system conspires to increase rather than decrease activity, and there are many contexts where this may be inappropriate. For example, it is not uncommon for older people to be on more than ten different drugs to treat an assortment of diseases and prevent others. The risks of harmful interaction rise exponentially and, with more than five drugs, have a high chance of harm occurring. This is a useful example of the modern mindset, which treats individual diseases as if they are independent of each other. In this context, drugs are given to prevent adverse outcomes – as if this were safer than not adding yet another drug to the list of those to be taken. This is an issue rarely discussed with much conviction in the medical press although individual GPs, and their patients and patients' relatives, are concerned and confused.

'Less' is not just beneficial from the perspectives of ecology and the economy but also, and crucially, in terms of health itself: less poly-pharmacy for older patients, less multiphasic screening, and so on. The disease factory model of the hospital would benefit by a shift towards a twenty-first-century version of the 'house of healing' (using insights from palliative care and elsewhere). Decreasing some forms of care, where clinically appropriate, will also release resources for where they are most needed and to address unmet need. It should be emphasized that this is *not* an argument for service rationing or reduction on the grounds of economic or any other instrumental aim. One way of expressing this in ethical terms is to understand that health care is currently practised from a defensive ethic; an alternative might be a creative ethic. A defensive ethic multiplies activity in order to prevent litigation, whereas a creative ethic is one in which the inner resources of practitioner and patient are both brought to the interaction. Patient autonomy and agency are fully acknowledged in such an ethical perspective.

The second foundational principle of conventional ethics – that of autonomy – accordingly needs a new and relational emphasis: one that focuses on releasing those inner resources of practitioner and patient, and acknowledges the reciprocal dimension of that relationship. Modernity has emphasized the patient as a consumer with individual rights (Anderek 2007). True autonomy should rather lead to greater capacity for care of the self and others. Many in our modern specialized society have become deskilled and disempowered. Simple economics and the pressures of demographic change will make it not just desirable but inevitable that we develop new models based more on our capacity to provide self-care and mutual care. We should therefore make a virtue out of necessity, and promote a new manifestation of autonomy wherein people can seek help when needs dictate but lack neither the skills nor the confidence for self-care, when appropriate. The result of these two changes in emphasis will be a reduction in some types of health care, the emergence of greater capacity for self-care, mutual care and integrative care from the NHS and, potentially, the diminution of unwarranted forms of professional interference. Resources released by this change in emphasis could be used to address unmet needs where self-care is not possible.

4 Emergent and ecological ethics

A simple aim of policy should be to reduce the ecological footprint of the NHS. This could conceivably be achieved in several ways:

- First, pursue activities directed at energy efficiency, food procurement and equipment design. Many parts of the NHS are already beginning to explore these options.
- Second, abandon resource intensive policies that have marginal health gains (the disposable instrument culture is one example).

- Third, do some things differently. A very large proportion of acute care is directed towards patients who are in the last six to twelve months of their lives. Yet we have a default position which drives an approach to investigation and treatment that is resource intensive and often fails to serve the needs of the dying person.
- Fourth, do less, where appropriate. We may have to accept that in a resource-constrained world, we could be satisfied with less: fewer consultations, less treatment, less of some forms of health care. This does not mean that outcomes would automatically worsen; they could well improve.
- Fifth, simplify the NHS. The future is likely to be characterized by what is currently called 'downshifting' – voluntarily making life simpler with less choice and fewer demands. The NHS could embrace this philosophy and release the creativity of staff and patients so that a model for practice emerges which is not only simpler but leads to better outcomes and patient and practitioner satisfaction.
- Sixth, make every NHS facility accessible on foot, by bicycle, and by public transport.
- Seventh, produce drugs and equipment with as little reliance on petrochemicals as possible; all consumables used by the NHS should be produced locally where possible.
- Eighth and last, the NHS should acknowledge and act on broader ecological principles of 'contraction and convergence' (Meyer 2000) in the service of global social justice.

In addition, rather than speaking of the NHS as an abstract reality, it might be better framed as staff, patients, teams, services, facilities and so on, all working with the personal intention to leave the world in a better shape than we found it. This is a restorative ethic, relational and intrinsically more resilient than our current just-in-time delivery style.

5 Current aesthetics

The emerging NHS environment will be a healing environment. The meaning and purpose of an NHS building should be reflected in its physical manifestation (CABE 2009). Is it too much to imagine healing and care in the context of green spaces and beautiful but ergometric design? The NHS will be efficient in a new kind of way – a way that lifts the spirits and is 'beautiful' in the sense of being aesthetically satisfying. The core purpose of this is to enhance healing change and emergent integrative processes, which could be achieved by promoting the idea that all professionals are inherently creative. That is, we are all 'artists of our lives' in the sense that we can live creatively and are imbued with individual creativity that we wish to bring to the work environment.

We create in order to make life, work, and even the experience of suffering, meaningful. The barriers to realizing this vision are perhaps imaginative rather than financial, in an organizational culture where 'value for money' – although obviously important – tends to dominate other considerations.

6 Emergent and ecological aesthetics

The process of working for the NHS or experiencing care in the context of the NHS should foster a growth in consciousness, empathy and compassion, thus enhancing an enabling and integrative approach. Staff should be sustained in this, both by their daily practice and the culture of the whole working community. Continuing professional development (CPD) should promote human, humane and ecological insights as well as keeping us abreast of relevant factual/scientific developments. Training should cover the integrated application of all six domains of the framework shown in Figure 10.1. All professional work would consciously integrate 'the good, the true and the beautiful'.

Are we close to this framework?

The NHS does, increasingly, try to follow evidence-based practice so it has strengths in the dimension of current science, shown in Figure 10.2. However, part of our critique is that the pursuit of this dimension to the near exclusion of the other five is unhelpful, even dangerous. In the contemporary NHS we find few signs of dimension 2 (emergent and ecological science): little systems science or consideration of order generating rules, and scant insights from disciplines like anthropology, cognitive biology and the environmental sciences. The NHS does have a commitment to ethical practice and governance procedures (dimension 3 of the framework in Figure 10.2). Nonetheless, it can be accused of failing to promote deeper patient autonomy and creating too much iatrogenic disease (such as hospital acquired infections and some of the effects of poly-pharmacy, especially in older patients). These can be seen as symptomatic of the way the system is currently organized, perhaps even a price paid for its power.

As far as dimension 4 (ecological ethics) is concerned, the NHS still has a throw-away culture where narrow ideas of the financial bottom line drive most decisions, which in turn tends to drive out the human dimension from which the system derives much of its positive effect. Ecological ethics receive insufficient consideration and the conceptual work of considering how ecological and other emerging ethical concerns might impact on the NHS has yet to be completed.

Finally, the NHS arguably performs least well at present in dimensions 5 and 6 – the aesthetic dimensions of the framework. Conventional aesthetics hardly feature at all and we do not believe that many NHS workers feel able to fully bring their own self into their work, far less express their creativity. The idea that working for the NHS (or, for that matter, encountering it as a patient) might mobilize inner forms of consciousness (deep personal reflection, and so on) is far from the ethos of the current NHS. Individual practitioners probably know something of the power of mobilizing inner responses in their patients, but their working environment is unlikely to encourage this. There are, perhaps, some honourable exceptions to this with regard to the aesthetics of the built environment and the emergence of different, more integral philosophies of care exemplified in the development of the 'Maggie's Centres' for cancer care in the UK (Heathcote and Jencks 2010) and the King's Fund project on enhancing the healing environment (King's Fund 2010).

Does anyone else do it better?

Increasingly large numbers of patients are turning to complementary and alternative therapies (CAMs), which have a greater commitment to the art of care and the creation of healing environments. In short, they are strong on dimension 5 of the framework – current aesthetics. However, they are weak on dimension 1 (conventional science and its evidence base) and have probably not fully engaged in what we have called the emerging ecological dimensions (2, 4 and 6) in this framework.

The hospice movement is strong on dimensions 1 (evidence-based practice) and 3 (traditional ethics). Hospices tend to be more able than other parts of the NHS to promote autonomy and the ethic of doing no harm. They also pay great attention to beauty and the therapeutic environment – dimension 5 of Figure 10.2. So, the NHS may have something to learn from the hospice movement, although it is deeply ironic that patients may have to wait until their final illness before experiencing an integrated form of care. However, the hospice movement, like CAMs, has yet to really address dimensions 2, 4 and 6 of Figure 10.2. It has not yet begun to grapple with the 'change of age' we all face, and what it may mean for their work in future.

There is a small health care organization in Alaska called the South Central Foundation which embodies all six dimensions of our framework. This health care system, called the Nuka system of care (nuka being an indigenous word for large, strong, living structures) provides care to the indigenous Alaskan population and is funded by the federal government, therefore not so different from the publically-funded NHS. After two years of consultation with the indigenous Alaskan community, the organization set about intentionally designing a system of health care based on shared responsibility, a commitment to quality, and family wellness. At its heart lies the recognition that health care is primarily a human system. To reflect indigenous values, the relationships between staff and patients (called 'customer owners' in their system) and between staff had to change. Buildings are designed using traditional shapes and materials. The community are involved in a continuous dialogue with the organization. After a decade and a half, the organization can demonstrate radical improvements in healthcare outcomes, client and staff satisfaction and reduced use of hospital care, thus remaining affordable and sustainable.

Conclusion

The central dilemma is that the logic of the arguments rehearsed above may be sound but the prospects for such radical change seem, at present, implausible. If an integral approach was advocated via political and/or managerial means, the probable response from both patients and practitioners would be one of profound distrust. Massive change can only be catalyzed by informed professional leadership but would also, and crucially, require endorsement and leadership from the general population. We have merely begun to sketch out what the future NHS might look like, in response to the challenges of sustainability and our current ingenuity gap. We believe that people everywhere have an intuitive understanding of 'the true, the good and the beautiful', and an inherent ability to integrate these in their day-to-day personal lives. Yet those of us who work in the UK health system may find ourselves in a context that largely inhibits the expression of that intuitive understanding and inherent ability. The future NHS would look very different if underpinned by integrative principles and perspectives: it would have internalized the challenges of the modern diseases as well as conventional disease; it would have adopted an ecological perspective and a genuine commitment to social justice, at local and global levels. It would be a living system, created by the interactive responsibilities of staff and patients and their families. And it would work with staff and patients to raise their aspirations (where possible) and inspire individual and collective transformative change.

There is much else that needs to be said and done if a new transformational approach to health care in the UK and other affluent, post-industrial nations is to become a reality. The current system with its constant growth in expenditure and activity will have to change, both because it is doing (unintended) harm and is unsustainable across many dimensions (Hannah 2010). It will take a change in the culture of health care to change the system of health care. Mobilizing the inner resources inherent in each of us could transcend the shortcomings of the existing system, which will in turn mobilize the healing resources of individuals, communities and systems so powered.

Transformational (cultural and individual) change will help to release this resource but health care practitioners will undoubtedly need supportive and participatory processes to help them make this transition.

References

Alexander, B. (2008) *The Globalisation of Addiction: A Study in Poverty of the Spirit.* New York: Oxford University Press.

Anderek, W. (2007) From patient to consumer in the medical marketplace. *Cambridge Quarterly of Healthcare Ethics*, 16(1): 109–13.

Capra, F. (1997) *The Web of Life: A New Scientific Understanding of Living Systems.* New York: Anchor Books.

CABE (Commission for Architecture and the Built Environment) (2009) *Future Health: Sustainable Places for Health and Well-being*. London: CABE.

Foresight Report (2007) *Tackling Obesities – Future Choices: Project Report*. London: Government Office for Science.

Gleick, J. (1987) *Chaos: Making a New Science*. New York: Penguin Books.

Hannah, M. (2010) Costing an arm and a leg: a plea for radical thinking to halt the slow decline and collapse of the NHS. Aberdour: International Futures Forum. http://www.internationalfuturesforum.com/iff_publications.php?go=dl&id= 33&file_ref=xcemkjmkvo (accessed 16 September 2011).

Heathcote, E. and Jencks, C. (2010) *The Architecture of Hope: Maggie's Cancer Care Centres*. London: Frances Lincoln Ltd.

James, O. (2008) *The Selfish Capitalist*. London, Vermilion.

Jones, R.H. (2000) *Reductionism: Analysis and the Fullness of Reality*. London: Associated University Press.

King's Fund (2010) *Enhancing the Healing Environment: Reading List*. London: King's Fund.

Lane, R.E. (2000) *The Loss of Happiness in Market Democracies*. London: Yale University Press.

Meyer, A. (2000) *Contraction and Convergence: The Global Solution to Climate Change*. Totnes: Green Books.

Roberts, B. (2005) *The End of Oil*. London: Bloomsbury.

11 A fifth wave for public health and the future public health practitioner

Public health and worldviews

In the modern world we have created, we appear to behave as if organizations do the work, regardless of human capacities, consciousness, energy, passion and effort. The existing change model might be summarized as: get the organizations and programmes right and change will happen. Much public happiness may be diminished for a lack of care, attention and understanding as increasingly ineffective bureaucratic arrangements enter a round of tighter and tighter regulation/re-organization in futile attempts to effectively manage an increasingly complex world (Kegan 1994). A sense of unease and dissatisfaction is pervasive. Calls for an ecological public health illustrate other pervasive ecological concerns. Although this 'new' public health could successfully fuse traditional approaches with the sustainability agenda, it is unlikely to be a sufficient response (Hanlon and Carlisle 2010).

The central argument of this book has been that change is needed to move us beyond the technical and reductionist mindsets that have characterized modernity and produced our current ingenuity gap (Homer-Dixon 2000). In Chapter 9 it was suggested that, to rise to the challenges it faces, the future public health discipline will need to become integrative, ecological, ethical, creative, beautiful, embodied and reflexive. The future public health practitioner will also need to embody these qualities. Achieving transformational change of worldview for a discipline and its practitioners may seem inherently implausible. Yet a moment's reflection reminds us that the worldview of people who lived 500 years ago was radically different from our own. Indeed, those who lived only a century ago would find aspects of our current worldview unimaginable.

Should we not therefore anticipate equally radical change as we move into the future, hard though this may be to imagine? If we as public health professionals are to become integral, ecological, embodied, creative, ethical and reflexive in our worldview and practice, then we will need to draw on techniques and approaches that help us develop a fuller sense of who we are, and our relationship to the world around us. This should not be dismissed as a call to navel-gazing introspection which might divert energy from other urgent tasks but a much-needed opportunity to pause, reflect and re-think such questions and to develop a new worldview (Eckersley 2011).

As human beings, we create our worldviews through our everyday encounters with the world (Berger and Luckmann 1966). Children in any society learn to pick up certain signals as having more meaning and significance than others: this is how we all acquire language, social skills, observational abilities and cultural competence. This process is reinforced and maintained in adulthood, creating a dynamic through which individuals in a particular culture sustain and reproduce that culture. This works fine in stable conditions, when people are growing up and living in a society that has fixed roles and traditions and certain ways of knowing and being: in that cultural milieu, they feel 'at home'. Through this process, each culture generates its own distinct worldview. A pertinent example of this comes from work by a psychologist who showed photographs of an aquarium to groups of Asian and Anglo-European students and asked them to describe what they saw (Nesbitt 2003). Western students pointed out separate objects in the tank, whilst Asian students saw the whole tank and described the relationships between the objects within it. Neither group is right or wrong in terms of what they observe: they simply have different worldviews and mindsets. The future public health practitioner will need to understand how different perspectives are profoundly influential in shaping the ways in which all of us understand and act in the world.

How worldviews change

The issues outlined above can be used to consider the unfolding of human societies, where cultural transitions generate changes of worldview. To explore this further, it may be illustrative to consider how people's lives changed over the course of the four previous waves of public health interventions described in Chapter 2 – their outer social and cultural worlds and their ideas, mindsets and inner world.

- People living prior to and during the time of the very earliest stages of the first wave of public health development were still influenced to some extent by the pre-modern, largely feudal economy. Their inner world was dominated by Christian symbols and ideas: in Britain, the pre-modern sense of morality and ethics, of what is 'right', came almost solely from the Church and its teachings. The Church shaped culture while the feudal system determined the economy and social hierarchy. Nevertheless, in the society found during the first two waves of public health development, that which was understood as 'true' (the scientific), 'good' (the ethical) and 'beautiful' (the aesthetic) were still differentiated and able to develop, unconstrained by hegemonic forces such as religious beliefs or feudal systems.

• The Enlightenment and the first Industrial Revolution saw the emergence of one of the first generations for whom scientific understandings of life were acceptable, although it took the era that saw the second and third waves of public health for this to become fully established. People still attended church but may also, in thoughtful moments, have wondered how the Bible could be both incontrovertibly 'true' *and* compatible with new discoveries of the world. Many experienced stirrings of independent thought and the belief that people needed some freedom in deciding what is right and wrong. At the same time, the aesthetic dimension of life had opportunities to develop and diversify. People may still have enjoyed the music of church services, but they also flocked to the newly popular music hall. They may still have read the Bible (or at the very least been familiar with it as a text) but the new novels of the time also attracted mass audiences.

• As the third wave of public health merged into the fourth (round about the middle of the twentieth century), we can conceive of how the inner and outer world were both changing by imagining the life of a young social worker in a local council. In that social worker's own lifetime, science has expanded its influence enormously, in some instances morphing into an ideology best called 'scientism'. (Under scientism what really matters is that which is known empirically, can be supported by evidence, can be counted or measured and above all, can be shown to be value for money.) Even though she cannot easily articulate a critique of scientism and modernity, the social worker feels the force of this change. Targets dictate most priorities and there is little flexibility to respond to the individual needs of clients. Many members of staff in her organization feel like cogs in a machine: reorganizations occur almost every year and people feel alienated from their roles and their clients. Absenteeism is rising. Some resent the people they are trying to help because they fail to cooperate with programmes being measured by management, using 'metrics' as the sole means of determining success. Outside work, many people experience individualism, materialism and consumerism as normal parts of life.

The above examples of differing worldviews are used here to suggest that human nature is not fixed: rather, humans are able, when obliged by life conditions, to adapt to their environment by constructing new, more complex conceptual models of the world that allow them to handle new problems. Each age of our history has been characterized by an inner world which acts as an organizing principle, expressed through self-propagating ideas, habits, or cultural practices (Tarnas 1991). The objective world of structures, resources and economies interacts with this complex dynamic: new technologies, energy regimes, economic models, and class hierarchies arise out of inner worlds and cultures but also help to create and mould them (Bauman 2000).

The worldview of the Middle Ages is now unfamiliar to many living in 'modern' rather than 'traditional' societies. This is the world of authoritarian religion, which is absolutist (in the sense that it seeks to control all aspects of life) and demands obedience to codes, laws and rules that dictate morality. We see this worldview in fundamentalist forms of religion today. The worldview of modernity developed with the scientific and industrial revolutions. This has been a rationalistic worldview, where the self is expressed calculatedly, to reach goals and objectives. The emergence of a late modern worldview is also discernible, one that is relativistic in morals, arts and science. This worldview is more accepting of diversity and more egalitarian than those which preceded it. We see many manifestations of this worldview in today's public health. This is positive, but is it enough?

An emerging worldview

The worldviews that have dominated the recent history of the West (and the 'developed' North of the globe) conceptualize the world as a place made especially for humans and a place without limits: our task is to subdue and exploit the earth. This perspective arose out of a synthesis of the Christian creationist theology and the rationalistic ideas of the Enlightenment (Tarnas 1991). Many have viewed this synthesis as progress and compared themselves favourably with other forms of society, where peoples with different (i.e. non-scientific and non-rational) belief systems were often categorized as 'primitive'. For example, Andrew Jackson, one of the early US Presidents, openly appealed to the benefit of settling the United States with 'modern' people who would bring progress, factories and commerce, in contrast to the 'backward' indigenous peoples who inhabited the continent prior to colonization.

Social and behavioural scientists argue that none of us can experience 'reality' directly: our understandings are mediated by and constructed from our own interpretations of what we perceive, and our experience (Berger and Luckman 1966). As a result, each of us exists in a personal world of meaning which can be put at risk from inconvenient truths. To ensure that we are not overwhelmed by the uncertainty inherent in living in a world we can never truly know, we may choose to shut out such discomforts. The problem is that our own worldview encourages us to believe ourselves 'right' in holding this perspective, and to reject others. This is certainly the case with authoritarian forms of religion and narrow forms of rationalism but it is also applicable to the contemporary pluralistic, relativistic worldview, which nevertheless views its own non-judgemental perspective as more valid than others. However, unlike post-modernist analyses which insist that we have no basis for making value judgements between different worldviews, the future public health practitioner will need to be empathetic to each *and* aware of the need to move beyond these. We will need to develop not just a worldview that is compatible with our needs as human beings but an outer world that is compatible with the needs of our ecosystem (Cafaro 2001).

We can best do this not by saying there are no criteria with which to make judgements: rather, we can take a perspective on all worldviews that is respectful *and* critical, one that enables us to develop a deeper consciousness of the world around us and greater empathy for others. In one sense, this is simply an integral part of human nature. An increasingly deep level of consciousness and a wider circle of empathy is part of healthy development in each individual as he or she grows from infancy to adulthood. Babies have little or no awareness of the world into which they are born: they are concerned primarily with the satisfaction of their own immediate needs. The infant will, if healthy, outgrow this phase of development to become a toddler, a child, an adolescent, a young adult and so on. Each stage transcends and includes the stage before. Failure to navigate one of the stages of development can have severe consequences later. For example, failure of bonding or attachment with a parent can impede healthy development, hamper the ability to form empathetic relationships and may lead to poorer mental health in later life. Another example is when lack of employment or alternatives to employment make it difficult for adolescents to find a place in the adult world: antisocial behaviour, teenage pregnancy, gang culture and much else can result.

Society needs to ensure that there are effective means to ensure that all children pass safely through all stages of development, and that adults are also supported as they make their own transitions in life. The need for support in traversing many stages of development is a lifelong process. Family, kinship groups and the broader society through a variety of structures like schools, workplaces and clubs have historically provided these support structures. In the past, religious beliefs and institutions also played important roles. It is commonplace to observe that many of these supports have been eroded. What we need now are ways to rebuild some of what we have lost and the inventiveness to create new structures, where appropriate. The future public health and its practitioners have a vital role to play in this (Hanlon et al. 2010, 2011).

Developing a fifth wave for public health

In this section of the chapter, the focus turns to the development of a fifth wave for public health and its practitioners. The framework set out in Chapters 9 and 10 suggests that the future public health and its practitioners will need to retain much that remains positive in our disciplinary tradition while developing new insights, capacities, ways of thinking, understanding and acting. What follows is a brief sketch that illustrates the positive future which we need to move towards:

- **Individual health** will become a resource for living (WHO 1986) and health will be seen as an individual and collective responsibility as mutual dependence becomes a more obvious feature of society. An emphasis on the so-called 'early years' will be increasingly evident, as it is now well understood that intrauterine influences and interactions in the first two years of life determine a great deal of health in later life. The evidence base for effective interventions during these early years is likely to grow and society will come to value every child as an important member of society. Maintaining healthy working lives will also be seen as of strategic importance to society as well as of benefit to individuals and their families.

  Given the inevitable ageing of all global populations, healthy ageing will be an important public health objective. Freedom from disease and disability is already a major focus but to this will be added strategies to slow the decline of physiological systems and to maintain immunity and morphology. A lifelong commitment to maintaining strength, endurance, flexibility, speed, balance and agility will be part of people's resource for living.

- **Individual self-responsibility** will assume a new role. Anyone who has worked in public health is familiar with two main debates about this. On one side we have those who argue that we have to start by changing the material distribution of wealth and reforming our structures (class, education, business and so on), and this should be the focus of health improvement. The counter argument often comes from those who say 'the only thing we can change is ourselves'. From this perspective, change comes through transformed individuals rather than transformed structures. An integral approach to future public health practice could transcend this dichotomous debate. Currently, individuals are encouraged to change their lifestyles in a manner that can reflect victim blaming at worst (Crawford 1977) or the trivial motivations offered by social marketing and 'nudge' strategies (Thaler and Sunstein 2008) at best.

The future public health needs to do more to support human agency, motivated by a transformation of worldview while working to change social structures and culture. Public health will, therefore, balance its historical emphasis on physical disease prevention and health damaging behaviours with an engagement that fosters individual reflection, allied to concern for others and for the planet on which we all depend. Key to this will be activities that foster self-awareness and a sense of belonging. The individually-oriented public health agenda will be as concerned with fostering purpose, hope, motivation, vision, creativity and raised consciousness as it will be with, for example, healthy eating and exercise.

- At the level of **systems and society** sustainability in resource use will be a central concern. Society will use less 'stuff' and create much less waste (including CO_2). The importance of health will be reflected by health-promoting buildings and infrastructure, and institutions that nurture people. Laws and regulations will promote the 'good society' in balance with protecting the rights of the individual. The economy will, in time, put people before money: in short, economism will no longer hold sway. There will be greater equality in wealth, income and opportunity. Family and other structures that influence human relationships will be more nurturing.
- **Collectively** we will foster good interpersonal relationships, high trust and cooperation, mutual awareness and acceptance, social justice and strong ethical principles. Ethics arises from empathic concern for others. Evidence now suggests that human beings are more cooperative and sociable in nature than they are competitive and individualistic. The ability to feel what another is experiencing (empathy) is an intrinsic part of our humanity and is the basis for authentic, inner-directed morality (as opposed to adherence to externally imposed rules).

The above may well be viewed as utopian: we freely concede this charge. But it also represents a new vision of public health. In reality, we are unlikely to achieve transformational change in the absence of such a vision, a new conceptualization of what it means to practise public health. Worse, the lack of a positive vision may encourage dystopian views of the future or keep us stuck in the world of diminishing returns and the ingenuity gap (Homer-Dixon 2000). To begin to move in this new direction of travel we need to:

- recognize that the public health community is dealing not with simple systems that can be predicted and controlled, but complex adaptive systems with multiple points of equilibrium that are unpredictably sensitive to small changes within the system;

- rebalance our mindset: from 'anti' (antibiotics, war on drugs, combating inequalities) to 'pro' (well-being, balance, integration), and from dominion and independence (through specialist knowledge and expertise) to greater interdependence and cooperation (the capacity to learn from and with others);
- rebalance our models: from a mechanistic understanding of the world and of ourselves as mechanics who diagnose and fix what is wrong with individual human bodies or communities, to organic metaphors where we understand ourselves as gardeners, enabling the growth of what nourishes human life and spirit, and supporting life's own capacity for healing and health creation;
- rebalance our orientation: integrate the objective (measurement of biological and social processes) with the subjective (lived experience, inner transformation) and inter-subjective (shared symbols, meanings, values, beliefs and aspirations);
- develop a future consciousness to inform the present, enabling innovation to feed the future rather than prop up the current unsustainable situation; develop different forms of growth beyond the economic to promote high levels of human welfare;
- iterate and scale up through learning – a design process where we try things out, learn and share this learning. The major challenge of 'scaling up', which requires us to develop promising new approaches, should be taken as a natural process of growth, driven by a desire to adapt and learn, rather than a mechanistic process that managers in large bureaucracies have responsibility for rolling out.

Who will do this work?

During the first wave of public health when newly industrialized societies were struggling with their change of age, it was noted that the people involved in the work of public health were diverse and none of them were formally qualified in public health (because formal qualification had not been invented). It seems likely that something analogous might emerge in the future. Indeed, many of the key players may not consider themselves to be involved formally in public health at all: their influence on health will be a product of their primary intent. This is perhaps best illustrated by a real world example, shown in Box 11.1. The point is that Arvind is a public health worker with no mention of these words in his job title or objectives. What is being argued here is that the future public health will require an enormous workforce, but many of those who make the most important contributions will probably not see themselves as public health workers. Nonetheless, there will still be a need for a skilled public health workforce to give the whole endeavour energy and direction.

Box 11.1 Parivartan

Arvind Kejriwal worked as a civil servant in the revenue department of the Indian government but realized that most of the corruption in the system came from poor flows of information between government and citizens. In 2000 he took a sabbatical from his job to found the organization now known as Parivartan. He began, with others, to campaign for the establishment of right to information legislation to address inequities caused by blocks to the flow of information from government departments to citizens. A national right to information act was passed by the government of India in 2005. Arvind resigned from his post in 2006 and now works full time for Parivartan. Parivartan uses the Right to Information Act, alongside traditional forms of music and dance to engage in conversation with slum dwellers about their conditions and action to improve this. A typical session begins with the playing of drums and singing of songs with lyrics describing the problem as an introduction to a discussion about slum improvement.

Parivartan often produces official documents at such meetings to illustrate claims by government departments about how much they have spent in that slum on improvements – road and drain building, electricity installation or fresh water pumps. In most instances local residents can testify that the claimed works have never been carried out. While this description seems rather prosaic on the page, the effect of such insight in the slum is electric. Government requisition orders are passed round the crowd to those who can read who verify that the order suggests that improvements in the slum to roads, lighting and water supply have been carried out at some expense, when one can clearly see that this is not so. The organization owns no vehicles, has no air-conditioned offices or any of the trappings which one would normally associate with this kind of voluntary activity. Yet a wide range of volunteers continue to help and the impact on the lives (and the health) of some of India's poorest and least healthy residents is very real.

This work is in its early stages and, while life is not a problem to be solved, the human resources which Arvind has unlocked begin to show that another world, in which truth, good and beauty are redefined by the many, is possible.

Training a new workforce

What skills will the new public health workforce require? The short answer is: all the current skills and more. The curriculum for training the public health workforce is well known: one only needs to examine what is taught on a Masters of Public Health (MPH) course. There are underpinning sciences like epidemiology and biology, and the social and behavioural sciences, such as economics, sociology and psychology. There are key skills, such as management, research, project management, health needs assessment, health impact assessment, and so on. There are also more specialized areas, such as health protection and health improvement. So the typical MPH curriculum is already very large. Yet we also need insights from systems and ecological sciences, and the practice that flows from them. If students and practitioners are overwhelmed as it is, how likely are we to cope successfully with this additional load?

The curriculum stands in need of rethinking and renewal. While a basic understanding of its core disciplines will always be needed, the future public health practitioner will also need to balance this knowledge with a practice derived from immersion in the real-life struggles of communities. This will require skills in dialogue, facilitation and social learning. Immersion allows practitioners to discover the inter-dependencies of complex systems and how these interact to generate a picture of health, as well as discovering the multiple perspectives that people will have on any particular challenge. It requires patience, deep listening and a willingness to be open to new learning. With this wider perspective, the practitioner is less concerned to define problems but rather to frame them, setting them in a historical, cultural and socio-psychological context (Schön 1984). The skilled practitioner of the future will participate with others to create and synthesize health-creating, rather than health-destroying, ecologies.

Achieving transformational change

Yet still more is needed. Some have argued that, in order both to survive as a species and grow in complexity, humanity must adopt a new image of what it means to be human (Csikszentmilhalyi 2004). This will involve rediscovering a reward system beyond the material as the comfortable environments that we have created, believing that this will improve our lives, now undermine the essence of what makes life worth living (Csikszentmihalyi 2004). Recent re-conceptualizations of what it means to be human express awareness that greed and sex are not the only human characteristics necessary for survival: we need, and can demonstrate, cooperation and altruism (Clark 1998). This is not just wishful thinking, or irrelevant to the future public health. Recent developments in neuroscience and other disciplines underpin the contention that human consciousness has evolved throughout history and is continuing to do so. It has also been persuasively argued that this evolution has been triggered, at various times in our history, by the convergence of new revolutions in communication with new systems of energy use (Rifkin 2009). This convergence has worked to create ever more complex societies that in turn expanded human consciousness and – crucially – our capacity to empathize with others.

The comparatively recent discovery of mirror neurons demonstrates the neurophysiology of empathy. In simple terms, our experience of compassion for others (what Rifkin terms the 'circle of empathic involvement') widens when technology changes and society becomes more developed (Rifkin 2009). So, for example, during the dark ages in Europe most people used simple technologies and lived in small communities: their 'circle of empathy' was limited by their lack of contact with others, among other things. The development of the printing press, better sources of energy and improved agriculture helped facilitate the late humanist phase of the Renaissance and began the processes that led to modernity, which has been accompanied by a widening of human experience and an extension of the circle of empathy. But the development of increasingly complicated social, cultural and economic environments has each required a surge in energy use, which has led us relentlessly towards the depletion of natural resources. So the fundamental irony of human history – its central paradox – is that our growing empathic awareness of others has only been made possible by an ever-greater consumption of the Earth's resources, resulting in a dramatic deterioration of the health of the planet on which we all depend.

Our dilemma today can be described as a race between empathy and entropy. Can we develop our circle of empathy to include care for all human beings, all other living things and all ecosystems, before the entropy bill (in the form of our increasing effect on the planet) destroys us? If we are to do so, we will need a culture that fosters personal and collective growth, allied to forms of personal and professional practice, and new institutions, to support this. In such a culture, living creatively would become increasingly recognized as central to growth as would mutual awareness and acceptance. With this in mind, a new understanding of what it means to be human and the enlargement of the circle of empathy becomes a key aim for public health, because it is a crucial aim for us all.

The future public health

If we are to reduce inequalities and improve health and well-being while addressing gaps between the rich and poor of the world, then we require the synergistic interaction of the six dimensions of the integrative framework, at the levels of both public health leadership and daily practice. Equally, if public health practitioners are to be exemplars as well as advocates of what it means to live a 'healthy life' (in its fullest sense), this too becomes part of our practice. Public health work needs to integrate the science and art of practice, informed by an ethical vision. The approach explored in this book has encompassed the inner world of the individual, the material world of the physical body, the structures of our society, our cultural belief systems and values, and the relationship of all of these to the wider biosphere. It is concerned with theory and practice. Its approach is fundamentally about learning our way into the future. No one profession can lay claim to all of that territory, far less occupy and regulate it. Yet we will need dedicated people who understand how health is created and destroyed and have the skills and tenacity to work for positive change. In short, we will need the heirs to what we currently call public health professionals. These people will, however, be part of the enormous network or coalition that will be needed for the fifth wave, in a manner analogous to our first wave of development.

Human beings are capable of transformational change. Life must certainly have been challenging for our earliest ancestors in the African forests, when the climate changed and the grasslands spread, forcing them to find a new way to sustain themselves. Yet the hardship that forced our ancestors to learn how to survive on grassland led in time to migration and subsequent population of the rest of the world by early humans. Equally, it must have been difficult to develop agricultural techniques and the domestication of animals for the first time so that larger groupings of humans could be fed. We know, from the social histories and literature of the times, that it was profoundly difficult for agricultural workers across the UK to leave their way of life and learn to function as 'hands' in the factories and mills of the first Industrial Revolution. Yet each of these transitions represented an important chapter in human history. The challenge for the future public health – and for all of us – is to learn from past and present successes (and failures) and move beyond these to write the next chapter of this unfolding narrative. The public health community has a vitally important contribution to make to the many debates about the lives people want to lead, the societies we want to live in, and the futures we want to create.

References

Bauman, Z. (2000) *Liquid Modernity*. Cambridge: Polity Press.

Berger, P.L. and Luckmann, T. (1966) *The Social Construction of Reality: A Treatise in the Sociology of Knowledge*. Garden City, NY: Anchor Books.

Cafaro, P. (2001) Economic consumption, pleasure, and the good life. *Journal of Social Philosophy*, 32(4): 471–86.

Clark, M.E. (1998) Human nature: what we need to know about ourselves in the twenty-first century. *Zygon*, 33(4): 645–59.

Crawford, R. (1977) You are dangerous to your health: the politics and ideology of victim blaming. *International Journal of Health Services*, 7(4): 663–80.

Csikszentmihalyi, M. (2004) What we must accomplish in the coming decades. *Zygon*, 39(2): 359–66.

Eckersley, R. (2011) The science and politics of population health: giving health a greater role in public policy. *WebmedCentral: Public Health*, 2(3): WMC001697.

Hanlon, P. and Carlisle, S. (2010) Re-orienting public health: rhetoric, challenges and possibilities for sustainability. *Critical Public Health*, 20(3): 299–309.

Hanlon, P., Carlisle, S., Hannah, M., Reilly, D. and Lyon, A. (2011) Learning our way into the future public health: a proposition. *Journal of Public Health*, 33(3): 335–42.

Hanlon, P., Carlisle, S., Reilly, D., Lyon, A. and Hannah, M. (2010) Enabling well-being in a time of radical change: integrative public health for the 21st century. *Public Health*, 124: 305–12.

Homer-Dixon, T. (2000) *The Ingenuity Gap: Facing the Economic, Environmental, and Other Challenges of an Increasingly Complex and Unpredictable Future*. New York: Vintage Books.

Kegan, R. (1994) *In Over our Heads: The Mental Demands of Modern Life*. Cambridge, MA: Harvard University Press.

Nesbitt, R.E. (2003) *The Geography of Thought: How Westerners See Things Differently from Asians – And Why*. New York: Free Press.

Rifkin, J. (2009) *The Empathic Civilization: The Race to Global Consciousness in a World in Crisis*. Cambridge: Polity Press.

Schön, D. (1984) *The Reflective Practitioner: How Professionals Think in Action*. New York: Basic Books.

Tarnas, R. (1991) *The Passion of the Western Mind: Understanding the Ideas that Have Shaped our World*. New York: Random House.

Thaler, R.H. and Sunstein, C.R. (2008) *Nudge: Improving Decisions about Health, Wealth and Happiness*. New Haven, CT: Yale University Press.

World Health Organization (1986) *Ottawa Charter for Health Promotion*. Geneva: World Health Organization.

Index

Tables, boxes and figures are indicated by the relevant letter. For example 140F9.2 indicates figure 9.2 on page 140. Main coverage on a topic, such as a chapter, is indicated in bold, e.g. cultures **72–84.** Subheadings indicate more detailed entries.

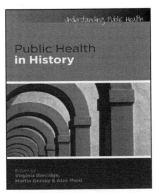

PUBLIC HEALTH IN HISTORY

Virginia Berridge, Martin Gorsky and Alex Mold

9780335242641 (Paperback)
2011

eBook also available

This fascinating book offers a wide ranging exploration of the history of public health and the development of health services over the past two centuries. The book surveys the rise and redefinition of public health since the sanitary revolution of the mid-nineteenth century, assessing the reforms in the post World War II years and the coming of welfare states.

Written by experts from the London School of Hygiene and Tropical Medicine, this is the definitive history of public health.

Key features:

- Case studies on malaria, sexual health, alcohol and substance abuse
- A comparative examination of why healthcare has taken such different trajectories in different countries
- Exercises enabling readers to easily interact with and critically assess historical source material

www.openup.co.uk

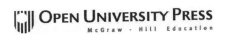

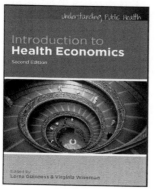

INTRODUCTION TO HEALTH ECONOMICS
Second Edition

Lorna Guinness and Virginia Wiseman

9780335243563 (Paperback)
September 2011

eBook also available

This practical text offers the ideal introduction to the economic techniques used in public health and is accessible enough for those who have no or limited knowledge of economics. Written in a user-friendly manner, the book covers key economic principles, such as supply and demand, healthcare markets, healthcare finance and economic evaluation.

Key features:

- Extensive use of global examples from low, middle and high income countries, real case studies and exercises to facilitate the understanding of economic concepts
- A greater emphasis on the practical application of economic theories and concepts to the formulation of health policy
- New chapters on macroeconomics, globalization and health and provider payments

www.openup.co.uk

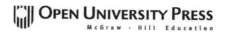

OPEN UNIVERSITY PRESS
McGraw - Hill Education

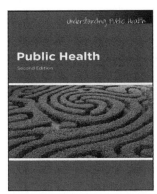

ISSUES IN PUBLIC HEALTH
Second Edition

Fiona Sim and Martin McKee

9780335244225 (Paperback)
September 2011

eBook also available

What is public health and why is it important? By looking at the foundations of public health, its historical evolution, the themes that underpin public health and the increasing importance of globalization, this book provides thorough answers to these two important questions.

Written by experts in the field, the book discusses the core issues of modern public health, such as tackling vested interests head on, empowering people so they can make healthy decisions, and recognising the political nature of the issues. The new edition has been updated to identify good modern public health practice, evolving from evidence

Key features:

- New chapters on the expanding role of public health, covering the issues of sustainability and climate change, human rights, genetics and armed conflict
- Examination of the impact of globalization on higher and lower income countries
- Expanded UK and International examples

www.openup.co.uk

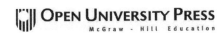

OPEN UNIVERSITY PRESS
McGraw - Hill Education